INTERMITTENT FASTING FOR HEALTHY LIFE

A Beginners Guide To Fit Your Body And
Follow Fasting Lifestyle With 21 Days
Diet Challenges and 10 Easy
Tips For success

Wayne K. Garrett

Table of Contents

3

DESCRIPTION

The concept of intermittent fasting is not new. Intermittent fasting is the process of avoiding food and calorie-rich drinks for a certain amount of time. Intermittent fasting or IF involves a cycle of eating and fasting. It is an eating pattern where one shift to periods of eating and fasting over a given period of time. There is nothing set in stone about it and you can do different types of intermittent fasting. Intermittent fasting isn't a diet. It is a way of eating that humans have been doing for centuries.

Don't confuse starvation with fasting. Fasting is completely different from starvation in one crucial way: control. Starvation is the involuntary abstention from eating. Fasting, on the other hand, is voluntary abstention from eating for health, weight loss, spiritual or other reasons. Food is readily available, but you choose not to eat it. Fasting has no standard duration. Anytime you are not eating and skipping meals are technically fasting.

This book has the best assortment of delicious, easy to make meals ranging from breakfast to desserts that will aid your weight loss within a short span of time. Are you ready? Grab this copy and start licking your fingers as you devour that luscious meal.

Happy cooking!

INTRODUCTION

When the body is forced to look for nourishment within itself rather than out, miraculous things happen. The human body acts as an anti-scarcity bank in times of food insecurity. Extra calories are kept inside the body stored as body fat or in the form of glycogen. And it is no understatement to say just how easy those extra calories come about. Just because you skip a few meals, it doesn't mean you suddenly die. Life is not a video game where you lose once you run out of lives or go hungry if you forgot to collect any food. The biochemical processes that govern the digestion of food and the delivery of usable energy to individual cells are much more complex. Very rarely are these processes explainable in terms of zero-sum games where once a resource is empty that is the end of the line. Instead, the body thrives on feedback loops, open systems and endogenous processes that work together to sustain life for as long as possible. These systems are so efficient that it is easy to mistake them for mere willpower. A world-class triathlete is able to push through a punishing amount of obstacles because their bodies are primed for that sort of thing. And though they are tired and constantly pushing themselves, their bodies work just as hard to allocate available resources and sustain their activity.

Thanks for downloading this book. It's my firm belief that it will provide you with all the answers to your questions.

BREAKFAST

01. Pizza Dip

Preparation Time: 15 minutes

Cook time: 22 minutes

Servings: 4

Ingredients:

- ¼ cup sour cream
- ½ cup mozzarella cheese
- 4 oz cream cheese, softened
- ¼ cup mayonnaise
- Salt and ground black pepper to taste
- ½ cup tomato sauce
- ¼ cup Parmesan cheese, grated
- 1 tbsp green bell pepper, seeded and chopped
- 6 pepperoni slices, chopped
- ½ tsp Italian seasoning
- 4 black olives, pitted and chopped

Directions:

1. In medium bowl, mix together sour cream, mozzarella cheese, cream cheese, mayonnaise, salt and pepper.

2. Put mixture into 4 ramekins.

3. Add in such orders: layer of tomato sauce, layer Parmesan cheese, chopped bell peppers, chopped pepperoni, Italian seasoning, chopped black olives.

4. Preheat oven to 350 F.

5. Place ramekins in oven and cook for 20 minutes. Serve.

Nutrition per Serving: Calories - 399, Carbs – 3.9g, Fat – 33.7g, Protein – 14.9g

02. Mexican Breakfast

Preparation Time: 15 minutes

Cook time: 32 minutes

Servings: 8

Ingredients:

- 1 lb chorizo
- 1 lb ground pork
- ½ cup enchilada sauce
- 8 medium eggs
- 3 tbsp butter
- Salt and ground black pepper to taste
- and chopped
- 4 oz onion, chopped
- 1 tomato, cored and chopped
- 1 avocado, pitted, peeled,

Directions:

1. Chop chorizo and mix well with ground pork.
2. Transfer mixture to baking sheet.
3. Top with enchilada sauce.
4. Preheat oven to 350 F.
5. Place baking sheet in oven and cook for 20 minutes.
6. In bowl, whisk eggs with salt and pepper.
7. Preheat pan over medium heat and melt butter.
8. Pour egg mixture in pan and cook slowly until eggs set, stirring now and then.
9. When pork mixture is cooked, place scrambled eggs over it.
10. Sprinkle with salt and pepper.
11. Top with onion, tomato and avocado. Serve.

Nutrition per Serving: Calories - 398, Carbs – 6.8g, Fat – 33g, Protein – 24.8g

03. Feta Omelet

Preparation Time: 12 minutes

Cook time: 11 minutes

Servings: 1

Ingredients:

- 1 tbsp heavy cream
- 3 eggs, beaten
- Salt and ground black pepper to taste
- 1 tbsp butter
- 1 oz feta cheese, crumbled
- 1 tbsp jarred pesto

Directions:

12. Whisk together heavy cream, eggs, salt and pepper.
13. Preheat pan over medium high heat and melt butter.
14. Pour in egg mixture and cook omelet until it's fluffy.
15. Sprinkle with cheese and pesto.
16. Fold omelet in half and cover pan. Cook for 5 minutes more.
1. Serve.

Nutrition per Serving: Calories - 497, Carbs – 3.1g, Fat – 44g, Protein – 29.5g

04. Creamy Scrambled Eggs

Preparation Time: 10 minutes

Cook time: 7 minutes

Servings: 1

Ingredients:

- 2 tbsp butter
- 4 large eggs, beaten
- 2 tbsp sour cream
- ½ tsp salt

- ¼ tsp black pepper
- 4 strips bacon
-

- 1 stalk green onion, chopped

Dircctions:

1. Preheat pan on medium heat and melt butter.

2. Add eggs and cook, stirring constantly.

3. When eggs are almost done, add sour cream and cook for 30 seconds more.

4. Sprinkle with salt and pepper and transfer to plate.

5. Add bacon strips to pan and let them cook for 1 minute on both sides.

6. Top eggs and bacons with green onion and serve.

Nutrition per Serving: Calories – 695, Carbs – 2.65g, Fat – 58g, Protein – 58.2g

05. Morning Pie

Preparation Time: 15 minutes

Cook time: 18 minutes

Servings: 4

Ingredients:

- 3 oz Parmesan cheese, sliced into thick pieces
- 5 medium eggs, beaten
- 8 oz full-fat cream cheese
- 4 cloves garlic, peeled

and minced
- 1 tsp salt
- ½ tsp cayenne pepper
- 1 tbsp butter
- 4 oz cream

Directions:

1. Put Parmesan cheese in baking form.

2. Place baking form in oven and cook for about 5 minutes on 360 F.

3. In medium bowl, whisk eggs. Add cream cheese and mix well.

4. In another bowl, combine garlic with salt and cayenne pepper.

5. Add garlic to egg mixture and stir well.

6. Heat up a pan, add and melt butter.

7. Pour egg mixture in pan and cook for 3 minutes on medium high heat, stirring constantly.

8. Place scrambled eggs on Parmesan cheese in baking form.

9. Top with cream and back baking form to oven. Cook for 10 minutes on 360 F.

10. Remove dish from oven and let it cool for about 10 minutes. Serve.

Nutrition per Serving: Calories - 389, Carbs – 4.9g, Fat - 34.7g, Protein - 18g

06. Blender Pancakes

Preparation Time: 10 minutes

Cook time: 12 minutes

Servings: 1

Ingredients:

- 2 large eggs, beaten
- 1 scoop vanilla protein powder
- 2 oz cream cheese
- 10 drops liquid stevia
- ¼ tsp salt

- 1/8 tsp cinnamon

Directions:

1. Place eggs, vanilla and cream cheese in blender or food processor and pulse it well.

2. Add liquid stevia, salt and cinnamon to food processor and blend until smooth.

3. Preheat pan on medium heat and spread pancake batter into 4-5" diameter rounds.

4. Bake on both sides until cooked.

5. Serve with sugar free maple syrup or butter.

Nutrition per Serving: Calories – 445, Carbs – 3.9g, Fat – 28.5g, Protein – 40.6g

07. Sausage Patties

Preparation Time: 15 minutes

Cook time: 12 minutes

Servings: 4

Ingredients:

- 1 lb minced pork
- Salt and ground black pepper to taste
- ½ tsp sage, dried
- ¼ tsp thyme, dried
- ¼ tsp ground ginger
- 3 tbsp cold water
- 1 tbsp coconut oil

Directions:

1. In small bowl, combine salt, sage, pepper, thyme, ginger and water.

2. In medium bowl, combine spice mix with pork.

3. Make patties and set aside.

4. Add coconut oil to pan and preheat it on medium high heat.

5. Transfer patties to pan and cook for 5 minutes, then flip, and cook them for 3 minutes more.

6. Serve.

Nutrition per Serving: Calories - 318, Carbs – 11g, Fat – 12.8g, Protein – 11.8g

08. Breakfast Mix

Preparation Time: 20 minutes

Cook time: 22 minutes

Servings: 6

Ingredients:

- 1 tsp turmeric
- ½ tsp oregano
- 1 tsp cilantro
- 1 tsp salt
- ½ tsp ground black pepper
- 1 tsp paprika
- 1¼ cup bacon, chopped
- 1 tbsp butter
- oz white mushrooms, sliced
- 1¼ cup zucchini, diced
- oz cauliflower, divided into florets
- oz asparagus, cut in half
- 2 cloves garlic
- 1 white onion, sliced
- 1 cup chicken broth

Directions:

1. In small bowl, mix together turmeric, oregano, cilantro, salt, pepper, and paprika.

2. Season bacon with spice mixture, stir well.

3. Heat up a pan, add and melt butter.

4. Add bacon to pan and cook for 5 minutes on medium heat, stirring constantly.

5. Add mushrooms, zucchini and cauliflower, stir and cook for another 2 minutes.

6. Stir in asparagus, garlic and onion and pour chicken broth.

7. Simmer for 10 minutes until vegetables are softened.

8. Serve warm.

Nutrition per Serving: Calories - 308, Carbs - 8.3g, Fat - 21.9g, Protein - 21g

09. Sausage Quiche

Preparation Time: 15 minutes

Cook time: 45 minutes

Servings: 6

Ingredients:

- 12 oz pork sausage
- 5 eggplants
- 10 mixed cherry tomatoes, halved
- 6 eggs, beaten
- 2 tsp whipping cream
- 2 tbsp Parmesan cheese, grated
- 2 tbsp fresh parsley, chopped
- Salt and ground black pepper to taste

Directions:

1. Chop sausage and place on the bottom of a baking dish.

2. Slice eggplants and lay on top.

3. Lay cherry tomatoes on eggplant.

4. In a medium bowl, combine eggs, cream, Parmesan cheese, parsley, salt and pepper.

5. Pour mixture over tomatoes.

6. Preheat oven to 375 F.

7. Place baking dish in oven and cook for 40 minutes.

8. Top with parsley and serve.

Nutrition per Serving: Calories - 338, Carbs – 2.9g, Fat – 27.5g, Protein – 17.1g

10. Sausage with Egg and Cheese

Preparation Time: 10 minutes

Cook time: 7 minutes

Servings: 1

Ingredients:

- 1 tsp olive oil
- 1 large egg, beaten
- 3 oz breakfast sausage, cooked
- 1 slice cheddar cheese
- Green onion, chopped (for garnish)

Directions:

1. Heat up pan with olive oil over medium heat, add eggs and fry until cooked (sunny side up or over easy).

2. Transfer to plate with cooked sausage and cheddar cheese.

3. Sprinkle with green onion and serve with your favorite hot sauce.

Nutrition per Serving: Calories – 404, Carbs – 1.1g, Fat – 42g,

Protein – 26g

11. Eggplant Stew

Preparation Time: 15 minutes

Cook time: 25 minutes

Servings: 6

Ingredients:

- 1 zucchini, sliced
- 1 cup chorizo sausages, sliced
- ½ tsp cayenne pepper
- 1 tsp basil
- 2 cups chicken broth
- 1 white onion, peeled and diced
- 1 cup eggplants, peeled and chopped
- 1 tbsp coconut oil
- 1 tsp salt

Directions:

1. In bowl, mix together zucchini and sausages.
2. Season with cayenne pepper and basil. Stir well.
3. Heat up pan and add chicken broth.
4. Add zucchini with sausages, onion, eggplant, and coconut oil.
5. Sprinkle with salt and stir.
6. Close lid and simmer dish for 20-25 minutes on medium heat.
7. After Cook stir carefully and serve.

Nutrition per Serving: Calories - 234, Carbs - 7g, Fat – 17.8g, Protein – 10.8g

12. Chicken Omelet

Preparation Time: 15 minutes

Cook time: 15 minutes

Servings: 1

Ingredients:

- 2 eggs, beaten
- Salt and ground black pepper to taste
- Olive oil spray
- 1 oz rotisserie chicken, cooked and shredded
- 1 tomato, cored and chopped
- 2 bacon slices, crumbled
- 1 small avocado, peeled and chopped
- 1 tbsp mayonnaise
- 1 tsp mustard

Directions:

1. In medium bowl, whisk together eggs, salt and pepper.
2. Preheat the pan on medium heat, add some Cook oil, pour in egg mixture and cook for 5 minutes.
3. Place chicken, tomato, bacon, avocado, mayonnaise and mustard on one half of omelet. Then fold omelet.
4. Close pan with lid and cook for about 5 minutes.
5. Serve warm.

Nutrition per Serving: Calories - 400, Carbs – 3.8, Fat – 31g, Protein – 26

13. Pepperoni Pizza Omelet

Preparation Time: 15 minutes

Cook time: 12 minutes

Servings: 1

Ingredients:

- Cooking spray
- 3 large eggs, beaten
- 1 tbsp heavy cream
- 4 oz pepperoni slices
- 4 oz mozzarella
- cheese, shredded
- Salt and ground black pepper to taste
- Dried basil to taste
- 2 bacon strips

Directions:

1. Preheat pan on medium heat and drizzle with cooking spray.

2. In bowl, combine eggs with heavy cream.

3. Pour mixture in pan and cook until almost done. Then add some pepperoni slices to one side.

4. Sprinkle cheese, black pepper, salt and basil over pepperoni and fold omelet over.

5. Cook for 1 minute more.

6. Meanwhile, in another pan fry bacon strips until cooked.

7. Serve omelet with cooked bacon.

Nutrition per Serving: Calories – 591, Carbs – 4.9g, Fat – 54g, Protein – 31.7g

14. Kale Fritters

Preparation Time: 15 minutes

Cook time: 10 minutes

Servings: 6

Ingredients:

- 7 oz kale, chopped (tiny pieces)
- 10 oz zucchini, washed and grated
- 1 tsp basil
- ½ tsp salt
- ¼ cup almond flour
- ½ tbsp mustard

- 1 large egg
- 1 tbsp coconut milk

- 1 white onion, diced
- 1 tbsp olive oil

Directions:

1. In medium bowl, mix together kale and zucchini.

2. Add basil and salt and stir.

3. Add almond flour and mustard. Stir well.

4. In another bowl, whisk together egg, coconut milk and onion.

5. Pour egg mixture into zucchini mixture and knead thick dough.

6. Preheat pan with olive oil on medium heat.

7. Shape fritters with help of spoon and put them in pan.

8. Cook fritters for about 2 minutes per side.

9. Transfer fritters to paper towel to remove excess oil.

10. Serve hot.

Nutrition per Serving: Calories - 120, Carbs – 8.8g, Fat – 8g, Protein - 5g

15. Italian Spaghetti Casserole

Preparation Time: 15 minutes

Cook time: 50 minutes

Servings: 6

Ingredients:

- 1 spaghetti squash, halved
- Salt and ground black pepper to taste

- 4 tbsp butter
- 2 cloves garlic
- 1 cup onion
- 4 oz tomatoes

- 3 oz Italian salami, chopped
- ½ cup Kalamata olives, chopped
- ½ tsp Italian seasoning
- 4 medium eggs
- ½ cup fresh parsley, chopped

Directions:

1. Heat up oven to 400 F.

2. Put squash on baking sheet. Sprinkle with salt and pepper.

3. Add 1 tablespoon butter and place in oven. Cook for 45 minutes.

4. Meanwhile, peel and mince garlic; peel and chop onion; core and chop tomatoes.

5. Preheat pan on medium heat, add and melt 3 tablespoons butter.

6. Add onion, garlic, salt and pepper, sauté for 2 minutes, stirring occasionally.

7. Add chopped tomatoes and chopped salami. Stir and cook for 10 minutes.

8. Add chopped olives and Italian seasoning. Stir and cook for 2-3 minutes more.

9. Remove squash halves from oven and scrape flesh with fork.

10. Combine spaghetti squash with salami mixture in pan.

11. Shape 4 spaces in mixture and crack egg in each.

12. Sprinkle with salt and pepper and place pan in oven.

13. Cook at 400 F until eggs are done.

14. Top with parsley and serve.

Nutrition per Serving: Calories - 328, Carbs – 11.9, Fat – 24g, Protein – 16

16. Cream Cheese Soufflé

Preparation Time: 15 minutes

Cook time: 20 minutes

Servings: 4

Ingredients:

- 1/3 cup spinach, chopped roughly
- 1 tsp coconut oil
- ¼ cup white onion, peeled and diced
- 1 egg, beaten
- ½ cup cream cheese
- ¼ cup coconut flour
- 1 tsp salt
- 1 tsp paprika

Directions:

1. Place spinach in blender or food processor and blend until texture smooth.
2. Preheat pan with coconut oil on medium heat.
3. Add onion and sauté for about 5 minutes, stirring constantly, until onion turn golden brown.
4. In medium bowl, combine egg, cream cheese and coconut flour.
5. Season mixture with salt and paprika, stir well.
6. Add cooked onion to mixture and stir.
7. Pour soufflé in baking dish.
8. Place dish in oven at 365 F and bake for 10 minutes
9. Remove baking dish from oven and whisk it carefully. Serve.

Nutrition per Serving: Calories - 196, Carbs - 5.3g, Fat – 16.9g, Protein - 5.6g

17. Morning Casserole

Preparation Time: 20 minutes

Cook time: 25 minutes

Servings: 4

Ingredients:

- 3 eggs, beaten
- 8 oz ground chicken
- 1 tsp salt
- 1 tsp oregano
- ½ tsp dried basil
- 1 tsp dried cilantro
- ½ tsp cayenne pepper
- 2 green bell peppers, deseeded and chopped
- 1 and 1/3 cup cauliflower, divided into florets
- 1 tbsp olive oil
- 6 oz Cheddar cheese, grated

Directions:

1. In medium bowl, combine eggs with chicken.
2. Season mixture with salt, oregano, basil, cilantro and cayenne pepper. Stir well.
3. In another bowl, mix together bell peppers and cauliflower.
4. Grease baking dish with olive oil.
5. Add chicken mixture to baking dish, lay cauliflower mixture on top, and sprinkle with Cheddar cheese.
6. Cover baking dish tightly with aluminum foil.
7. Place form in oven at 360F and cook for 10 minutes.
8. Remove foil and bake dish for another 10 minutes.
9. Remove baking dish from oven and let it cook for 5-7 minutes. Serve.

Nutrition per Serving: Calories - 229, Carbs - 5.4g, Fat - 16g,

Protein - 17.8g

18. Breakfast Bread

Preparation Time: 12 minutes

Cook time: 5 minutes

Servings: 4

Ingredients:

- 1 egg, beaten
- ⅓ cup almond flour
- 2½ tbsp coconut oil
- ½ tsp baking powder
- A pinch of salt

Directions:

1. Whisk together egg, almond flour, oil, baking powder and salt.
2. Grease a microwave-safe form with some coconut oil.
3. Pour egg mixture into form and place in microwave.
4. Cook for 3 minutes on high heat.
5. When bread is cooked, let it cool for 5-10 minutes.
6. Slice and serve.

Nutrition per Serving: Calories - 119, Carbs – 2.8g, Fat – 11.8g, Protein – 4.2g

FISH & SEAFOOD

19. Wrapped and Grilled Salmon with Saffron

Serves: 4

Preparation Time:10 minutes

Cooking: 10 minutes

Ingredients

- 3/4 cup black olives, pitted and cut into quarters

- 1 grated tomato

- 1/4 cup olive oil

- 2 cloves fresh garlic minced

- 1/2 tsp sea salt and freshly ground black pepper to taste

- 1 tsp fresh thyme finely chopped

- Pinch of saffron (15 to 20 threads)

- 4 salmon fillets

Directions

1. Preheat your grill (pellet, gas, charcoal) to HIGH according to manufacturer instructions.

2. In a medium bowl, combine all ingredients (except salmon).

3. Set one piece of salmon on foil and sprinkle lightly with salt and pepper. Spoon a quarter of the mixture over the fish and seal the foil tightly. Repeat to make four packets.

4. Place on the grill, cover the lid and cook for about 8-10 minutes. Transfer fish packets on a serving plate, and allow it to cool before serving.

Nutrition per Serving: Calories: 361 Carbohydrates: 4.6g 32g Proteins: Fat: 4g Fiber: 1.4g

20. Creamy Tuna and Mushrooms Casserole

Serves: 5

Preparation Time:10 minutes

Cooking: 15 minutes

Ingredients

- 1/4 cup of olive oil

- 15 white mushrooms sliced

- 2 can (15 oz) tuna fish

- 1 1/4 cups of cream

- 1 1/4 cups of grated cheddar cheese

Directions

1. Preheat the oven to 400 F/200 C.
2. Heat the oil in a large skillet over high heat.
3. Add the mushrooms and sauté for two minutes.
4. Add the tuna fish and cream; gently stir.
5. Pour the tuna mixture in a heat-proof dish and sprinkle with grated cheese.
6. Bake for 15 minutes or until bubbling. Serve hot.

Nutrition per Serving: Calories: 551 Carbohydrates: 3g Proteins: 51g Fat: 38g Fiber: 0.5g

21. Lemon Salmon and Broccoli Casserole

Serves: 4

Preparation Time:10 minutes

Cooking: 15 minutes

Ingredients

- 1 Tbsp of olive oil
- 1 onion finely chopped
- 1 cup of mushrooms
- 1 large broccoli
- 2 cloves garlic
- 1 lb smoked salmon
- 1 cup of cream
- 3/4 cup of water
- Lemon juices of 2 lemons
- Capers, to taste
- 1 cup of grated cheese

Directions

1. Heat the olive oil in a large over-proof saucepan over medium heat and sauté the onions and mushrooms for 2 - 3 minutes.
2. Add the garlic and broccoli, cook, stirring occasionally, for a total of 5 minutes.
3. Add water and cream, and season with the salt and pepper.
4. Add the lemon juice and mix.
5. Add the cream, smoked salmon and capers and mix again.
6. Cover with the grated cheese and put in the oven, broil about 3 minutes, while the cheese is melted.

Nutrition per Serving: Calories: 503 Carbohydrates: 8.5g Proteins: 34g Fat: 38g Fiber: 1g

22. Herbed Shrimp with Cilantro

Serves: 6

Preparation Time:15 minutes

Cooking: 4 minutes

Ingredients

- 1 cup water

- 1 1/2 lb large shrimp, peeled

- 1 bunch cilantro, finely chopped

- 1/4 cup olive oil

- 1 cup grated tomato

- 2 cloves garlic, minced

- 1 tsp cumin

- 1 tsp coriander

- 1 tsp turmeric

- 3 Tbsp of lime juice, freshly squeezed

Directions

1. Pour water to the inner stainless steel pot in the Instant Pot.

2. Add shrimp and sprinkle with chopped cilantro and pinch of salt.

3. In a bowl, stir together the olive oil, grated tomato, garlic, cumin, coriander and turmeric.

4. Pour the mixture over shrimp and cilantro; toss to combine well.

5. Lock lid into place and set on the MANUAL setting for 3 -4 minutes.

6. When the timer beeps, press "Cancel" and carefully flip the Quick Release valve to let the pressure out.

7. Serve hot shrimp with sauce.

Nutrition per Serving: Calories: 168 Carbohydrates: 2.5g Proteins: 16g Fat: 13g Fiber: 0.5g

23. Seafood - Coconut Stew

Serves: 8

Preparation Time:10 minutes

Cooking: 2 minutes

Ingredients

- 1 lb white fish fillet
- 2 pinch of sea salt
- 2 cloves garlic, finely chopped
- 1 Tbsp coriander fresh, finely chopped
- 1 lemon juice, freshly squeezed

- 2 Tbsp olive oil
- 2 spring onions finely chopped
- 1 grated tomato
- 1 lb of shrimp
- 2 cups of coconut milk
- 1 cup water

Directions

1. Season the fish with salt, garlic, coriander and lemon juice.
2. Pour olive oil in your Instant Pot and layer the fish fillets.
3. Put chopped onions, tomatoes and peppers and sprinkle with a coriander on top.
4. Pour 1/2 cup water.
5. Lock lid into place and set on the MANUAL setting for 2 minutes.
6. When the timer beeps, press "Cancel" and carefully flip the Quick Release valve to let the pressure out.
7. Open the lid and add shrimps and coconut milk: stir to combine well.
8. Lock lid into place and set on the MANUAL setting for 1 minute.

9. Use Quick Release - turn the valve from sealing to venting to release the pressure.

10. Serve hot.

Nutrition per Serving: Calories: 221 Carbohydrates: 4g Proteins: 21g Fat: 15g Fiber: 0.5g

24. Simple "Grilled" Shrimp

Serves: 4

Preparation Time:10 minutes

Cooking: 2 minutes

Ingredients

- 2

- Tbsp fresh butter softened

- 1 1/2 lb shrimp (21-25 size, peeled, deveined)

- Sea-salt flakes

- 1 Tbsp fresh tarragon and chervil finely

chopped

- 1 cup water

- Lemon wedges for serving

Directions

1. Add the butter to the inner stainless steel pot in the Instant Pot.

2. Add shrimp into Instant Pot, and sprinkle with sea-salt flakes and chopped tarragon and chervil.

3. Lock lid into place and set on the MANUAL setting for 2 minutes.

4. When the timer beeps, press "Cancel" and carefully flip the

Quick Release valve to let the pressure out.

1. Ready! Serve with lemon wedges.

Nutrition per Serving: Calories: 62 Carbohydrates: 4g Proteins: 1g Fat: 6g Fiber: 3g

25. Mussels ala Marinera

Serves: 6

Preparation Time:15 minutes

Cooking: 3 hours

Ingredients

- 4 lbs of mussels, cleaned
- 1 small onions, chopped
- 1 Tbsp of ground paprika
- 2 Tbsp of almond flour
- 1 glass of white wine
- 1 cup of bone broth
- A bunch of chopped fresh parsley
- Salt to taste
- 2 Tbsp of extra virgin olive oil
- 6 bay leaves

Directions

1. Place the mussels in your Slow Cooker along with all remaining ingredients.
2. Cover and cook on HIGH for 2 hours.
3. Open lid, remove mussels; debeard and clean them.
4. Place mussels in a Slow Cooker, cover and cook on HIGH for further 1 hour.

5. Serve.

Nutrition per Serving: Calories: 310 Carbohydrates: 7g Proteins: 42g Fat: 8g Fiber: 0.2g

26. Temptation Shrimp in Sauce

Serves: 6

Preparation Time:5 minutes

Cooking: 3 hours and 40 minutes

Ingredients

- 3
- cloves garlic, pressed
- 1/2 cup olive oil
- 2 bay leaves
- 1 1/2 cup white wine
- 1/4 tsp Salt
- 1/2 tsp of cayenne powder
- 1/4 cup Tabasco sauce (optional)
- 1 fresh lemon juice
- 3 Tbsp Worcester sauce
- 1 Tbsp Fresh parsley, chopped
- 1 Tbsp of fresh rosemary leaves
- 3 lbs fresh whole shrimps

Directions

1. Combine all ingredients (except shrimp) in your 6- or 8-quart Slow Cooker.
2. Cover and cook on LOW for 2 - 3 hours.
3. Open lid and add shrimp in Slow Cooker; toss to combine well with the sauce.

4. Cover and cook on HIGH heat for 30 -40 minutes or until shrimp are pink.

5. Serve shrimp with cooking sauce.

Nutrition per Serving: Calories: 165 Carbohydrates: 5g Proteins: 3g Fat: 12g Fiber: 0.5g

27. Coconut Aminos Shrimps Stir-fry

Serves: 4

Preparation Time:10 minutes

Cooking: 15 minutes

Ingredients

- 2 lbs medium shrimp
- 3 Tbsp coconut aminos (from coconut sap)
- 1 lemon zest
- 1/2 cup lemon juice (freshly squeezed)
- for garnish
- 2 Tbsp of olive oil
- 2 green onions (finely chopped)
- Salt and freshly ground pepper
- 2 Tbsp fresh coriander leaves finely chopped

Directions

1. In a bowl, whisk the coconut aminos, lemon juice and zest, and the salt and pepper.

2. Place shrimp in a large container and cover with coconut aminos sauce; cover and refrigerate for 2 hours.

3. Heat the oil in a large frying skillet.

4. When hot, sauté the green onion for 5 - 6 minutes.

5. Add marinated shrimps and stir-fry for 3 - 3 1/2 minutes (for

large 3 - 4 minutes).

6.   Garnish with coriander and serve hot.

Nutrition per Serving: Calories: 245 Carbohydrates: 5g Proteins: 32g Fat: 10g Fiber: 1.5g

28. Grouper Fish and Celery Casserole

Serves: 8

Preparation Time:10 minutes

Cooking: 15 minutes

Ingredients

- 3 1/2 lbs of grouper fish (or swords, sea bass)
- 1 1/2 lb of fresh celery chopped
- 1/2 cup white wine
- 1 cup of olive oil
- Salt and black pepper freshly ground
- Juice of 1 lemon juice

Directions

1.   Season the fish with the salt and pepper.
2.   Rinse and clean the celery and finely cut.
3.   Place the celery in a large saucepan.
4.   Place the fish slices over celery.
5.   Pour the olive oil, lemon juice and wine; cook over high heat until boil.
6.   Reduce the heat to medium, cover and cook for 5-6 minutes.
7.   Taste and adjust salt and pepper to taste.

8. Serve hot.

Nutrition per Serving: Calories: 371 Carbohydrates: 3.4g Proteins: 23g Fat: 29g Fiber: 1.55g

29. Shrimp, Fish, and Fennel Soup

Serves: 6

Preparation Time:10 minutes

Cooking: 15 minutes

Ingredients

- 2 Tbsp garlic-infused olive oil
- 1 scallion, green parts only, chopped
- 1 fennel bulb, finely sliced
- Salt and ground white pepper
- 1 tomato, peeled and grated

- 1/4 cup fresh parsley, finely chopped
- 1 Tbsp fresh coriander leaves, finely chopped
- 4 cups water
- 12 oz of medium shrimp
- 12 oz of cod fillets
- 2 Tbsp lemon zest

Directions

1. Heat the oil in a large pot over medium-high heat.
2. Sauté the scallion and sliced fennel until softened.
3. Season the scallion with the salt and ground white pepper.
4. Add the parsley and coriander; pour the water and bring to boil; cook for 5 minutes.
5. Add grated tomato and cook for 2 - 3 minutes; stir.

6. Add the cod fish and shrimp, and simmer for further 4 - 5 minutes.

7. Taste and adjust seasonings.

8. Serve hot.

Nutrition per Serving: Calories: 112 Carbohydrates: 4g Proteins: 12g Fat: 6g Fiber: 2.2g

30. Baked Sea Bass with Fresh Herbs

Serves: 4

Preparation Time:10 minutes

Cooking: 20 minutes

Ingredients

2 Tbsp extra virgin olive oil

1 tsp fresh thyme chopped

1 tsp garlic, finely chopped

- 1 tsp fresh mint finely chopped
- 1/2 Tbsp fresh basil chopped
- 1/2 tsp sea salt and ground black pepper
-
- to taste
- 4 fillets Sea bass skinless
- Lemon slices for serving
- Olive oil for greasing

Directions

1. Preheat the oven to 400F/200C. Grease with the olive one baking dish; set aside.

2. In a small bowl, combine together a thyme, mint, basil, garlic, salt and pepper and stir well.

3. Apply the herb mixture and rub on both sides of fish fillets.

4. Place the fish fillets in prepared baking dish.

5. Bake for 20 minutes or until done.

6. Serve warm and garnish with lemon slices.

Nutrition per Serving: Calories: 308 Carbohydrates: 1g Proteins: 46g Fat: 12g Fiber: 1g

CHICKEN & POULTRY

31. One Pan Chicken Mix

Preparation time: 10 minutes

Cooking time: 16 minutes

Servings: 4

Ingredients:

- 1 and ½ pounds chicken thighs, boneless and skinless
- 2 teaspoons thyme, chopped
- A pinch of salt and black pepper
- 1 tablespoon olive oil
- 12 ounces Brussels sprouts, halved
- 1 red onion, sliced
- 1 garlic clove, minced
- 2 teaspoons stevia
- 2 tablespoons balsamic vinegar
- 1/3 cup walnuts, chopped

Directions:

1. Heat up a pan with the oil over medium-high heat, add chicken pieces, season with salt, pepper and thyme, cook for 5 minutes on each side and transfer to a plate.
2. Heat up the same pan over medium-high heat, add Brussels sprouts, garlic and onion, stir and cook for 6 minutes.
3. Add stevia and vinegar, stir and take off heat.
4. Divide the chicken between plates, add Brussels sprouts in the side and sprinkle walnuts on top.
5. Enjoy!

Nutrition per Serving: Calories 231, fat 4, fiber 7, carbs 12, protein 25

32. Chicken Chili

Preparation time: 10 minutes

Cooking time: 20 minutes

Servings: 6

Ingredients:

- 1 pound chicken, ground
- 2 garlic cloves, minced
- 1 yellow onion, chopped
- 1 and ½ tablespoon olive oil
- 1 tablespoon chili powder
- 7 ounces canned green chilies, chopped
- 28 ounces canned tomatoes, chopped
- 3 cups butternut squash, peeled and cubed
- 14 ounces chicken stock
- A pinch of salt and black pepper

Directions:

1. Heat up a pot with the oil over medium-high heat, add chicken, garlic and onion, stir and cook for 6 minutes.
2. Add chili powder, chilies, tomatoes, squash, stock, salt and pepper, stir, cover the pot, simmer for 15 minutes, divide into bowls and serve.
3. Enjoy!

Nutrition per Serving: Calories 211, fat 3, fiber 4, carbs 13, protein 7

33. Chipotle Chicken

Preparation time: 10 minutes

Cooking time: 12 minutes

Servings: 4

Ingredients:

- 1 pound chicken breast, skinless, boneless and cut into strips
- 1 teaspoon chili powder
- 1 teaspoon cumin, ground
- A pinch of salt and black pepper
- 1 tablespoon olive oil
- 1 red bell pepper, sliced
- 1 cup mushrooms, sliced
- 1 yellow onion, chopped
- 1 tablespoon chipotles in adobo sauce, chopped
- 3 garlic cloves, minced
- 1 and ½ tablespoons lime juice

Directions:

1. Heat up a pan with the oil over medium-high heat, add chicken strips, chili powder, cumin, salt and pepper, stir and cook for 6 minutes.

2. Add bell pepper, mushrooms, onion, chipotles, garlic and lime juice, stir, cook for 6 minutes more, divide into bowls and serve.

3. Enjoy!

Nutrition per Serving: Calories 212, fat 3, fiber 6, carbs 15, protein 18

34. Chicken and Tomatoes

Preparation time: 10 minutes

Cooking time: 16 minutes

Servings: 4

Ingredients:

- 4 chicken breast fillets, skinless and boneless
- A pinch of salt and black pepper
- 1 tablespoon olive oil
- ¼ cup parmesan, grated
- , halved
- 1 tablespoon parsley, chopped
- 1 garlic clove, minced
- 1 pound cherry tomatoes

Directions:

1. Grease a baking dish with the oil, add chicken fillets, tomatoes and garlic, season with salt and pepper, sprinkle parmesan and parsley, introduce in the oven and cook for 16 minutes at 450 degrees F.
2. Divide everything between plates and serve.
3. Enjoy!

Nutrition per Serving: Calories 251, fat 3, fiber 6, carbs 11, protein 13

35. Chicken, Squash and Apples

Preparation time: 10 minutes

Cooking time: 40 minutes

Servings: 3

Ingredients:

- 1 butternut squash, peeled and cubed

- 2 tablespoons olive oil

- 1 apple, cored and cubed

- 2 chicken breasts, skinless and boneless

- 1 tablespoon cilantro, chopped

- A pinch of salt and pepper

Directions:

1. In a bowl, mix squash with apples, cilantro, salt, pepper and 1 tablespoon oil and toss.

2. Heat up a pan with the rest of the oil over medium heat, add chicken, salt and pepper and cook for 5 minutes on each side.

3. Add apple and squash mix, stir, introduce everything in the oven at 425 degrees F and bake for 20 minutes.

4. Shred the meat, divide everything between plates and serve.

5. Enjoy!

Nutrition per Serving: Calories 210, fat 14, fiber 3, carbs 11, protein 15

36. Chicken and Pineapple Mix

Preparation time: 10 minutes

Cooking time: 13 minutes

Servings: 4

Ingredients:

- 20 ounces canned pineapple, cubed

- 1 tablespoon olive oil

- A pinch of salt and black pepper

- 3 cups chicken thighs, boneless, skinless and cut into medium pieces

- 1 tablespoon sweet paprika

- 1 tablespoon cilantro, chopped

Directions:

Heat up a pan with the oil over medium-high heat, add chicken, salt, pepper and paprika, toss, cook for 10 minutes, add pineapple and cilantro, cook for 3 minutes more, divide everything between plates and serve.

Nutrition per Serving: Calories 220, fat 3, fiber 7, carbs 8, protein 12

37. Chicken and Mango Chutney

Preparation time: 10 minutes

Cooking time: 10 minutes

Servings: 4

Ingredients:

- 4 chicken breast halves, skinless and boneless

- 1 tablespoon coconut aminos

- 2 tablespoons lime juice

- 2 tablespoons olive oil

- 2 tablespoons mango chutney

- 1 cup mango, peeled and chopped

- 1 avocado, peeled, pitted and chopped

- A pinch of salt and black pepper

Directions:

1. In a bowl, mix the chicken with oil, chutney, lime juice, and coconut aminos and toss to coat.

2. Heat up your kitchen grill over medium-high heat, add chicken, reserve 1 tablespoon chutney mix, cook for 4 minutes on each side, cut into thin strips, put in a salad bowl, add mango, avocado and reserved chutney, toss and serve.

3. Enjoy!

Nutrition per Serving: Calories 210, fat 3, fiber 4, carbs 8, protein 15

38. Chicken and Cucumber Mix

Preparation time: 10 minutes

Cooking time: 0 minutes

Servings: 4

Ingredients:

- 2 chicken breast halves, cooked and shredded

- 2 cucumbers, cubed

- 4 green onions, chopped

- A pinch of salt and black pepper

- 3 tablespoons mustard

- ¼ cup mint, chopped

- 2 cups baby spinach

Directions:

1. In a bowl, mix chicken with cucumbers, onions, mint, spinach, mustard, salt and pepper, toss and serve.

2. Enjoy!

Nutrition per Serving: Calories 230, fat 4, fiber 4, carbs 8, protein 15

39. Chicken and Parsnips

Preparation time: 10 minutes

Cooking time: 40 minutes

Servings: 6

Ingredients:

- 1 whole chicken, cut into medium pieces
- 3 tablespoons olive oil
- Salt and black pepper to the taste
- 1 yellow onion, chopped
- 1 tablespoon black peppercorns, crushed
- 4 parsnips, sliced
- 1 cup celery, chopped
- 1 cup chicken stock
- 2 tablespoons parsley, chopped
- 4 carrots, sliced

Directions:

1. Heat up a pot with the oil over medium-high heat, add the chicken, brown it for 5 minutes on each side and transfer to a bowl.

2. Heat up the same pan over medium-high heat, add the onion, peppercorns, parsnips, celery and carrots, stir and cook for 5

minutes more.

3. Return the chicken pieces, also add the stock, cover and cook everything for 25 minutes more.

4. Add parsley, divide everything between plates and serve. And serve.

5. Enjoy!

Nutrition per Serving: Calories 250, fat 7, fiber 3, carbs 12, protein 9

40. Chicken and Leeks Mix

Preparation time: 10 minutes

Cooking time: 1 hour and 30 minutes

Servings: 4

Ingredients:

1. 1 whole chicken
2. A pinch of salt and black pepper
3. 1 cup veggie stock
4. 1 cup tomato sauce
5. 1 leek, sliced
6. 1 carrot, sliced
7. 3 tablespoons olive oil
8. 2 cups yellow onion, chopped
9. ½ cup lemon juice

Directions:

1. Grease a baking dish with the oil, add chicken, season with a pinch of salt and black pepper, add leek, carrots, onion, lemon juice, veggie stock and tomato sauce, toss, introduce in the oven and bake at 400 degrees F for 1 hour and 30 minutes.

2. Carve the chicken, divide it and the veggies between plates and serve with cooking juices on top.

3. Enjoy!

Nutrition per Serving: Calories 219, fat 3, fiber 5, carbs 6, protein 20

41. Indian Chicken Soup

Preparation time: 10 minutes

Cooking time: 2 hours

Servings: 5

Ingredients:

- 1 whole chicken, cut into medium pieces
- 1 yellow onion, chopped
- 3 and ½ quarts veggie stock
- 4 carrots, chopped
- 4 celery ribs, chopped
- 1 garlic clove, minced
- 1 teaspoon black peppercorns
- 6 parsley springs
- A pinch of salt and black pepper
- ¼ cup olive oil
- 2 tomatoes, chopped
- 2 tablespoons ginger, grated
- 1 tablespoon tomato paste
- 1 cup coconut milk
- 1 green banana, chopped
- 2 tablespoons cilantro, chopped

Directions:

1. Put chicken in a pot, add the stock, onion and carrots, stir and bring to a simmer over medium heat.

2. Add peppercorns, garlic and parsley springs, stir, cover and simmer for 1 hour and 30 minutes.

3. Meanwhile, heat up a pan with the oil over medium-high heat, add tomatoes, ginger, tomato paste and curry powder, stir and cook for 7 minutes.

4. Add banana and coconut milk, stir, and pour everything over the soup, cook for 30 minutes more, ladle into bowls, sprinkle cilantro on top and serve.

5. Enjoy!

Nutrition per Serving: Calories 219, fat 9, fiber 5, carbs 10, protein 9

42. Chicken and Almond Butter Stew

Preparation time: 10 minutes

Cooking time: 40 minutes

Servings: 4

Ingredients:

- 1 cup chicken stock
- 1 garlic clove, minced
- ½ yellow onion, chopped
- 8 ounces chicken breast skinless, boneless and chopped
- 1 cup collard greens, chopped
- ½ cup soft almond butter
- Salt and black pepper to the taste
- 2 tablespoons ginger, grated

Directions:

1. Put the stock in a pot, add garlic, chicken and onion, stir, bring to a boil over medium heat and simmer for 20 minutes.

2. In a bowl, mix almond butter with 1 tablespoon soup, stir well, and pour over the mix in the pot.

3. Add collard greens, salt, pepper and ginger, stir and cook for 5 more minutes.

4. Divide into bowls and serve.

5. Enjoy!

Nutrition per Serving: Calories 209, fat 5, fiber 5, carbs 8, protein 11

43. Chinese Chicken Soup

Preparation time: 15 minutes

Cooking time: 15 minutes

Servings: 4

Ingredients:

- 1 and ½ tablespoon five spice powder
- 3 chicken thighs boneless, skinless and cut into small pieces
- A pinch of salt and black pepper
- 2 tablespoons olive oil
- 1 chili pepper, chopped
- 2 garlic cloves
- 1 head bok choy, chopped
- 2 tablespoons coconut aminos
- ½ cup cilantro, chopped
- 3 cups chicken stock

Directions:

1. Put chicken in a bowl, season with salt, pepper and five spice powder and rub.

2. Heat up a pot with the oil over medium heat, add garlic and chili pepper, stir and cook for 3 minutes.

3. Add chicken, bok choy, aminos and stock, stir, cook for 12 minutes, divide into bowls and serve with chopped cilantro on top.

4. Enjoy!

Nutrition per Serving: Calories 227, fat 4, fiber 5, carbs 10, protein 9

44. Chicken and Bacon Soup

Preparation time: 10 minutes

Cooking time: 30 minutes

Servings: 4

Ingredients:

- 12 ounces chicken thighs, skinless, boneless and cubed

- 3 smoked bacon slices, chopped

- 1 cup tomato, chopped

- ½ cup yellow onion, chopped

- 1 garlic clove, minced

- 2 tablespoon oregano, chopped

- Salt and black pepper to the taste

- 3 cups veggie stock

- 2 tablespoons cilantro, chopped

Directions:

Heat up a pot over medium-high heat, add bacon, stir, cook for 7 minutes, take off heat and transfer to a bowl

Heat up the same pot over medium heat, add chicken, cook for 6 minutes, and put in the same bowl with the bacon.

Return the pot to medium heat one more time, add garlic and onion, stir and cook for 4 minutes.

Add tomato, salt, pepper, oregano, bacon, chicken and stock, stir, bring to a boil, cook for 6 minutes more, add parsley, stir, ladle into soup bowls and serve.

Enjoy!

Nutrition per Serving: Calories 205, fat 4, fiber 5, carbs 12, protein 26

BEEF, LAMB & PORK

45. Easy Pork Roast Casserole

Serves: 5

Preparation Time:10 minutes

Cooking: 1 hour

Ingredients

- 2 Tbsp butter
- 2 lbs of pork roast
- 1 green onion chopped
- 1 Tbsp of almond flour
- 1/2 cup of white wine
- 1 cup of bone broth
- 1/2 cup of cream
- 3 fresh tarragon sprigs
- 3 slices of Cheddar cheese
- Salt and ground pepper to taste

Directions

1. Heat the butter in a casserole over medium heat.
2. Brown the roast for 5 - 6 minutes, and add chopped green onion.
3. Pour the wine and let simmer for 2 - 3 minutes.
4. Season with the salt and pepper, pour the bone broth, cover and cook for 30 minutes.
5. Add the cream and chopped tarragon and gently stir.
6. Place cheddar slices on the top of meat, cover and cook for further 15 minutes.
7. Serve hot.

Nutrition per Serving: Calories: 549 Carbohydrates: 2g Proteins: 43.5g Fat: 40g Fiber: 0.1g

46. Pork and Bacon Baked Casserole

Serves:

Preparation Time:10 minutes

Cooking: 25 minutes

Ingredients

- 2 lbs pork loin cut large strips
- Salt and pepper to taste
- 1 Tbsp of lard
- 1/2 lb of bacon, finely chopped
- 1 spring onion finely chopped
- 2 cloves of garlic finely chopped
- 1 cup of white wine
- 3 bay leaves

Directions

1. Preheat oven to 350 degrees F/170 C.
2. Season the pork strips with the salt and pepper.
3. In a deep and heavy frying skillet, heat the lard over medium - high heat.
4. Fry the bacon for 2 minutes.
5. Add the green onion and garlic, and sauté for 2 - 3 minutes; stir.
6. Add the pork meat and season with the salt and pepper; stir for 2 minutes.
7. Pour wine, sprinkle with crumbled bay leaves, and season

with the salt and pepper.

8. Transfer the mixture in the casserole pan.

9. Place in oven and bake for 20 - 25 minutes. Serve hot.

Nutrition per Serving: Calories: 412 Carbohydrates: 2g Proteins: 38g Fat: 24g Fiber: 0.2g

47. Pork with Button Mushrooms Casserole

Serves: 4

Preparation Time:10 minutes

Cooking: 30 minutes

Ingredients

- 1 Tbsp of almond flour

- Salt and freshly ground black pepper

- 1 1/2 lbs of pork loin chops, cut in strips

- 2 Tbsp of butter

- 1 green onion, chopped

- 2 cloves of garlic, finely sliced

- 1 cup of button mushrooms

- 1 cup red wine

- 1/2 cup of water

- 1 tsp of fresh thyme

- 1 Tbsp of mustard grain

Directions

1. In a large container, combine the almond flour with thyme and the salt and pepper, and roll the pork strips.

2. Heat the butter in a large casserole dish over medium heat and sauté the pork for 2 - 3 minutes.

3. Add all remaining ingredients and sprinkle with the salt and

54

pepper; stir only for 2 - 3 minutes.

4.   Bake in a oven for about 20 minutes

5.   Serve hot.

Nutrition per Serving: Calories: 341 Carbohydrates: 5.5g Proteins: 40g Fat: 17g Fiber: 1g

48. "Kaula" Pork with Cabbage

Serves: 6

Preparation Time:15 minutes

Cooking: 5 minutes

Ingredients

- 3 lbs pork tenderloin
- 2 tsp garlic powder
- 1 Tbsp kosher salt
- 1/2 cup bone broth (preferable homemade)
- 1/2 cup of water
- 1 small head of cabbage cut in chunks

Directions

1.   Season salt and garlic powder over pork.

2.   Place the pork in your Instant Pot; pour bone broth and water.

3.   Lock lid into place and set on the MANUAL setting on HIGH pressure for 85 minutes.

4.   After the pressure cooking time has finished, use Natural Release - it takes 10 - 25 minutes to depressurize naturally.

5.   Open lid and remove the pork to a large bowl.

6. Add the cabbage wedges in your Instant Pot and sprinkle with the salt.

7. Lock lid into place and set on the MANUAL setting on HIGH for 3 minutes.

8. Use Quick Release - turn the valve from sealing to venting to release the pressure.

9. Place cabbage wedges on a large serving platter.

10. Use two forks and shred the pork. Spoon the pork over the cabbage, and pour with juice from the Pot.

Nutrition per Serving: Calories: 282 Carbohydrates: 6g Proteins: 50g Fat: 6g Fiber: 3g

49. Mouth-watering Shredded BBQ Roast

Serves: 8

Preparation Time:10 minutes

Cooking: 30 minutes

Ingredients

- 4 lbs pork roast

- 1 tsp garlic powder

- Salt and pepper to taste

- 1/2 cup water

- 2 can (11 oz) of barbecue sauce, unsweetened

Directions

1. Season the pork with garlic powder, salt and pepper; place in your Instant Pot.

2. Pour water and lock lid into place; set on the MEAT/STEW,

high pressure setting for 30 minutes.

3. When ready, use Quick Release - turn the valve from sealing to venting to release the pressure.

4. Remove pork in a bowl, and with two fork shred the meat.

5. Pour BBQ sauce and stir to combine well.

6. Serve.

Nutrition per Serving: Calories: 373 Carbohydrates: 2.5g Proteins: 34g Fat: 24g Fiber: 3g

50. Sour and Spicy Spareribs

Serves: 10

Preparation Time:15 minutes

Cooking: 35 minutes

Ingredients

- 5 lbs spare spareribs
- Salt and pepper to taste
- 2 Tbsp of tallow
- 1/2 cup coconut aminos (from coconut sap)
- 1/2 cup vinegar
- 2 Tbsp Worcestershire sauce, to taste
- 1 tsp chili powder
- 1 tsp garlic powder
- 1 tsp celery seeds

Directions

1. Cut the rack of ribs into equal portions.

2. Season salt and ground pepper your spare ribs from all sides.

3. Add tallow in your Instant Pot and place spare ribs.

4. In a bowl, combine together all remaining ingredients and

pour over spareribs.

5. Lock lid into place and set on the MANUAL setting on HIGH heat for 35 minutes.

6. When the timer beeps, press "Cancel" and carefully flip the Natural Release for 20 minutes.

7. Open the lid and transfer ribs on a serving platter.

8. Serve hot.

Nutrition per Serving: Calories: 598 Carbohydrates: 2g Proteins: 36g Fat: 54g Fiber: 0.2g

51. Tender Pork Shoulder with Hot Peppers

Serves: 8

Preparation Time:10 minutes

Cooking: 30 minutes

Ingredients

- 3 lbs pork shoulder boneless
- Salt and ground black pepper to taste
- 3 Tbsp of olive oil
- 1 large onion, chopped
- 2 cloves garlic minced
- 2 - 3 chili peppers, chopped
- 1 tsp ground coriander
- 1 tsp ground cumin
- 1 ½ cups of bone broth (preferable homemade)
- 1/2 cup water

Directions

1. Season salt and pepper the pork meat.

2. Turn on the Instant Pot and press SAUTÉ button. When the word "hot" appears on the display, add the oil and sauté the onions and garlic about 5 minutes.

3. Add pork and sear for 1 - 2 minutes from all sides; turn off the SAUTÉ button.

4. Add all remaining ingredients into Instant Pot.

5. Lock lid into place and set on the MEAT/STEW setting on HIGH heat for 30 minutes.

6. When the timer beeps, press "Cancel" and carefully flip the Natural Release button for 15 minutes. Serve hot.

Nutrition per Serving: Calories: 389 Carbohydrates: 2.5g Proteins: 36g Fat: 27g Fiber: 0.5g

52. Braised Sour Pork Filet

Serves: 6

Preparation Time:10 minutes

Cooking: 8 hours

Ingredients

- 1/2 tsp of dry thyme
- 1/2 tsp of sage
- Salt and ground black pepper to taste
- 2 Tbs of olive oil
- 3 lbs of pork fillet
- 1/3 cup of shallots (chopped)
- 3 cloves of garlic (minced)
- 3/4 cup of bone broth
- 1/3 cup of apple cider vinegar

Directions

1. In a small bowl, combine together thyme, sage, salt and black

ground pepper.

2. Rub generously pork from all sides.

3. Heat the olive oil in a large frying pan, and sear pork for 2 - 3 minutes.

4. Place pork in your Crock Pot and add shallots and garlic.

5. Pour broth and apple cider vinegar / juice.

6. Cover and cook on SLOW for 8 hours or on HIGH for 4-5 hours.

7. Remove pork on a plate, adjust salt and pepper, slice and serve with cooking juice.

Nutrition per Serving: Calories: 348 Carbohydrates: 3g Proteins: 51g Fat: 12.5g Fiber: 0.1g

53. Pork with Anise and Cumin Stir-fry

Serves: 4

Preparation Time:5 minutes

Cooking: 30 minutes

Ingredients

- 2 Tbsp lard
- 2 spring onions finely chopped (only green part)
- 2 cloves garlic, finely chopped
- 2 lbs pork loin, boneless, cut into cubes
- Sea salt and black ground pepper to taste
- 1 green bell pepper (cut into thin strips)
- 1/2 cup water
- 1/2 tsp dill seeds
- 1/2 anise seeds
- 1/2 tsp cumin

Directions

1. Heat the lard n a large frying pot over medium-high heat.

2. Sauté the spring onions and garlic with a pinch of salt for 3 - 4 minutes.

3. Add the pork and simmer for about 5 - 6 minutes.

4. Add all remaining ingredients and stir well.

5. Cover and let simmer for 15 - 20 minutes

6. Taste and adjust seasoning to taste. Serve.

Nutrition per Serving: Calories: 351 Carbohydrates: 3g Proteins: 1g Fat: 51.5g Fiber: 1g

54. Baked Meatballs with Goat Cheese

Serves: 8

Preparation Time:15 minutes

Cooking: 35 minutes

Ingredients

- 1 Tbsp of tallow
- 2 lbs of ground beef
- 1 organic egg
- 1 grated onion
- 1/2 cup of almond milk (unsweetened)
- 1 cup of red wine
- 1/2 bunch of chopped parsley
- 1/2 cup of almond flour
- Salt and ground pepper to taste
- 1/2 Tbsp of dry oregano
- 4 oz of hard goat cheese cut in cubes

Directions

1. Preheat oven to 400 F/200 C.

2. Grease a baking pan with tallow.

3. In a large bowl, combine all ingredients except goat cheese.

4. Knead the mixture until ingredients are evenly combined.

5. Make small meatballs and place in a prepared baking dish.

6. Place one cube of cheese on each meatball.

7. Bake for 30 - 35 minutes.

8. Serve hot.

Nutrition per Serving: Calories: 404 Carbohydrates: 2.2g Proteins: 25.5g Fat: 31g Fiber: 0.5g

55. Parisian Schnitzel

Serves: 4

Preparation Time:15 minutes

Cooking: 10 minutes

Ingredients

- 4 veal steaks; thin schnitzel

- Salt and ground black pepper

- 2 Tbsp of butter

- 3 eggs from free-range chickens

- 4 Tbsp of almond flour

Directions

1. Season steaks with the salt and pepper.

2. Heat butter in a large non-stick frying pan at medium heat.

3. In a bowl, beat the eggs.

4. Add almond flour in a bowl.

5. Roll each steak in almond flour, add then, dip in beaten eggs.

6. Fry about 3 minutes per side.

7. Serve immediately.

Nutrition per Serving: Calories: 355 Carbohydrates: 0.3g Proteins: 54g Fat: 15g Fiber: 0g

56. Beef Stroganoff

Serves: 6

Preparation Time:5 minutes

Cooking: 30 minutes

Ingredients

- 2 lbs of rump or round steak or stewing steak
- 4 Tbsp of olive oil
- 2 green onions, finely chopped
- 1 grated tomato
- 2 Tbsp ketchup
- (without sugar)
- 1 cup of button mushrooms
- 1/2 cup of bone broth
- 1 cup of sour cream
- Salt and black pepper to taste

Directions

1. Cut the meat into strips and sauté in large frying skillet.

2. Add chopped onion and a pinch of salt, and cook meat for about 20 minutes at medium temperature.

3. Add mushrooms and ketchup and stir for 3 - 5 minutes.

4. Pour the bone broth and sour cream, and cook for 3 - 4 minutes.

5. Remove from the heat, taste and adjust salt and pepper to taste.

6. Serve hot.

Nutrition per Serving: Calories: 348 Carbohydrates: 4,2g Proteins: 37g Fat: 21g Fiber: 1g

57. Meatloaf with Gruyere

Serves: 6

Preparation Time:15 minutes

Cooking: 40 minutes

Ingredients

- 1 1/2 lbs ground beef
- 1 cup ground almonds
- 1 large egg from free-range chickens
- 1/2 cup grated Gruyere cheese
- 1 tsp fresh parsley finely chopped
- 1 scallion finely chopped
- 1/2 tsp ground cumin
- 3 eggs boiled
- 2 Tbsp of fresh grass-fed butter, melted

Directions

1. Preheat oven to 350 F175 C.

2. Combine all ingredients (except eggs and butter) in a large bowl.

3. Using your hands, combine well the mixture.

4. Shape the mixture into a roll and place in the middle sliced hard-boiled eggs.

5. Transfer the meatloaf to a 5x9 inch loaf pan greased with melted butter.

6. Place in oven and bake for 40 minutes or until internal temperature of 160 degrees F.

7. Remove from the oven and allow rest for 10 minutes.

8. Slice and serve.

Nutrition per Serving: Calories: 598 Carbohydrates: 5,3g Proteins: 28g Fat: 63g Fiber: 2.6g

SALADS

58. Lunch Caesar Salad

Preparation Time: 15 minutes

Cook time: 0 minutes

Servings: 2

Ingredients:

- 1 avocado, pitted
- 1 chicken breast, grilled and shredded
- 1 cup bacon, cooked and crumbled
- 3 tbsp creamy Caesar dressing
- Salt and ground black pepper to taste

Directions:

1. Peel and slice avocado.
2. In medium bowl, combine bacon, chicken breast and avocado.
3. Add creamy Cesar dressing, stir well.
4. Season with salt and pepper, stir.
5. Serve.

Nutrition per Serving: Calories - 329, Carbs – 2.99g, Fat – 22.9g, Protein – 17.8g

59. Asian Side Salad

Preparation Time: 35 minutes

Cook time: 12 minutes

Servings: 4

Ingredients:

- 1 green onion
- 1 cucumber
- 2 tbsp coconut oil
- 1 packet Asian noodles, cooked
- ¼ tsp red pepper
- aste

- flakes
- 1 tbsp sesame oil
- 1 tbsp balsamic vinegar
- 1 tsp sesame seeds
- Salt and ground black pepper to t

Directions:

1. Chop onion. Slice cucumber thin.
2. Preheat pan with oil on medium high heat.
3. Add cooked noodles and close lid.
4. Fry noodles for 5 minutes until crispy.
5. Transfer noodles to paper towels and drain grease.
6. Combine cucumber, pepper flakes, green onion, sesame oil, vinegar, sesame seeds, pepper, salt and noodles. Mix well.
7. Put in refrigerator at least for 20-30 minutes. Serve.

Nutrition per Serving: Calories - 397, Carbs – 3.97g, Fat – 33.7g, Protein – 1.98g

60. Egg Salad

Preparation Time: 15 minutes

Cook time: 0 minutes

Servings: 4

Ingredients:

- 6 oz ham, chopped
- 5 eggs, boiled and chopped
- 1 tsp garlic, minced
- ½ tsp basil
- 1 tsp oregano
- 1 tbsp apple cider vinegar
- 1 tsp kosher salt
- ½ cup cream cheese

Directions:

1. In medium bowl, combine chopped ham with chopped eggs, stir.
2. In another bowl, mix together garlic, basil, oregano, vinegar, and salt. Stir the mixture till you get homogeneous consistency.
3. Whisk together spice mixture and cream cheese.
4. Add cream cheese sauce to egg mixture and stir gently.
5. Serve.

Nutrition per Serving: Calories - 341, Carbs – 4.99g, Fat - 26g, Protein – 22.1g

61. Cobb Salad

Preparation Time: 20 minutes

Cook time: 27 minutes

Servings: 1

Ingredients:

- 1 tbsp olive oil

- 4 oz chicken breast

- 2 strips bacon

- 1 cup spinach, chopped roughly

- 1 large hard-boiled egg, peeled and chopped

- ¼ avocado, peeled and chopped

- ½ tsp white vinegar

Directions:

1. Heat up pan on medium heat and add oil.

2. Add chicken breast and bacon, cook until get desired crispiness.

3. Add spinach and egg, stir.

4. Add avocado and mix well.

5. Sprinkle with white vinegar and stir.

6. Serve.

Nutrition per Serving: Calories - 589, Carbs – 2g, Fat – 47.8g, Protein – 42g

62. Bacon and Zucchini Noodles Salad

Preparation Time: 15 minutes

Cook time: 0 minutes

Servings: 3

Ingredients:

- 32 oz zucchini noodles

- 1 cup baby spinach

- ⅓ cup blue cheese, crumbled
- ½ cup bacon, cooked and crumbled
- ⅓ cup blue cheese dressing
- Ground black pepper to taste

Directions:

1. Combine zucchini noodles, spinach, blue cheese, and bacon, Stir carefully.
2. Add black pepper and cheese dressing, toss to coat. Serve.

Nutrition per Serving: Calories - 198, Carbs – 1.99g, Fat – 13.9g, Protein – 9.95g

63. Chicken Salad

Preparation Time: 15 minutes

Cook time: 0 minutes

Servings: 3

Ingredients:

- 1 celery stalk
- 2 tbsp fresh parsley
- 1 green onion
- 5 oz chicken breast, roasted and chopped
- 1 egg, hard-boiled, peeled and chopped
- Salt and ground black
- pepper to taste
- ½ tsp garlic powder
- ⅓ cup mayonnaise
- 1 tsp mustard
- ½ tbsp dill relish

Directions:

1. Wash and chop celery, parsley and onion.
2. Place celery, onion and parsley in blender or food processor and blend well.
3. Remove this mass from food processor and set aside.
4. Place chicken in food processor and pulse well.
5. Add chicken to onion mixture and stir.
6. Add egg, pepper and salt, stir gently.
7. Add garlic powder, mayonnaise, mustard and dill relish, toss to coat.
8. Serve.

Nutrition per Serving: Calories - 279, Carbs – 2.99g, Fat – 22.9g, Protein – 11.9g

64. Asparagus Salad

Preparation Time: 20 minutes

Cook time: 0 minutes

Servings: 5

Ingredients:

- 2 lbs asparagus, cooked and halved
- 1 tbsp butter, melted
- ½ tsp garlic powder
- 1 tsp sesame seeds
- 1 tbsp coconut oil
- 1 tbsp apple cider vinegar
- 1 tsp dried basil
- 1 tsp salt
- 4 oz Parmesan cheese, grated

Directions:

1. In bowl, combine asparagus, butter and garlic powder. Stir well.
2. Add sesame seeds, coconut oil, vinegar, basil and salt. Mix well.
3. Set salad aside to marinate.
4. Serve salad with grated Parmesan cheese.

Nutrition per Serving: Calories - 133, Carbs - 7g, Fat - 8.85g, Protein - 10g

65. Apple Salad

Preparation Time: 15 minutes

Cook time: 0 minutes

Servings: 4

Ingredients:

- 1 medium apple
- 2 oz pecans
- 16 oz broccoli florets
- 1 green onion
- 2 tsp poppy seeds
- Salt and ground black pepper to taste
- ¼ cup sour cream
- ¼ cup mayonnaise
- ½ tsp lemon juice
- 1 tsp apple cider vinegar

Directions:

1. Core and grate apple. Chop pecans and broccoli florets. Dice green onion.

2. In bowl, combine broccoli, apple, pecans, and green onion. Stir well.

3. Sprinkle with poppy seeds, black pepper and salt, stir carefully.

4. In another bowl, whisk sour cream, mayonnaise, lemon juice and vinegar.

5. Add this mixture to salad and toss to coat.

6. Serve.

Nutrition per Serving: Calories - 249, Carbs – 3.9g, Fat – 22.9g, Protein – 4.8g

66. Bok Choy Salad

Preparation Time: 20 minutes

Cook time: 10 minutes

Servings: 6

Ingredients:

- 10 oz bok choy, chopped roughly
- 2 tbsp coconut oil
- 4 tbsp chicken stock
- 1 tsp basil
- 1 tsp ground black pepper
- 1 white onion, peeled and sliced
- ¼ cup white mushrooms, marinated and chopped
- 1 lb tofu, chopped
- 1 tsp oregano
- 1 tsp almond milk

Directions:

1. Heat up pan on medium heat.

2. Add bok choy, 1 tablespoon of oil and chicken stock.

3. Season with basil and black pepper.

4. Add onion and close lid.

5. Simmer vegetables for 5-6 minutes, stirring constantly.

6. Transfer vegetables to bowl and add mushrooms.

7. Pour 1 tablespoon of oil in pan and heat it up again.

8. Add chopped tofu and cook for 2 minutes.

9. Transfer tofu to bowl with vegetables and sprinkle with oregano.

10. Pour in almond milk and toss to coat.

11. Serve salad.

Nutrition per Serving: Calories - 130, Carbs - 4.67g, Fat - 11g, Protein – 6.9g

67. Halloumi Salad

Preparation Time: 15 minutes

Cook time: 12 minutes

Servings: 2

Ingredients:

- 3 oz halloumi cheese, sliced
- 1 cucumber, sliced
- ½ cup baby arugula
- 5 cherry tomatoes, halved
- 1 oz walnuts, chopped
- Salt and ground black pepper to taste
- ½ tsp olive oil
- ¼ tsp balsamic vinegar

Directions:

1. Preheat grill on medium high heat.
2. Put halloumi cheese in grill and cook for 5 minutes per side.
3. In mixing bowl, combine cucumber, arugula, tomatoes, and walnuts.
4. Place halloumi pieces on top.
5. Sprinkle with black pepper and salt.
6. Drizzle oil and balsamic vinegar, toss to coat.
7. Serve.

Nutrition per Serving: Calories - 448, Carbs – 3.98g, Fat – 42.8g, Protein – 22.3g

68. Smoked Salmon Salad

Preparation Time: 17 minutes

Cook time: 0 minutes

Servings: 4

Ingredients:

- 8 oz smoked salmon, sliced into thin pieces
- 2 oz pecans, crushed
- 3 medium tomatoes, chopped
- ½ cup lettuce, chopped
- 1 cucumber, diced
- 1/3 cup cream cheese
- 1/3 cup coconut milk
- ½ tsp oregano
- 1 tbsp lemon juice, chopped
- ½ tsp basil
- 1 tsp salt

Directions:

1. In medium bowl, combine salmon with pecans and stir.

2. Add tomatoes, lettuce and cucumber, stir well.

3. In another bowl, mix together cream cheese, coconut milk, oregano, lemon juice, basil and salt. Stir mixture until get homogenous mass.

4. Serve salmon salad with cream cheese sauce.

Nutrition per Serving: Calories - 211, Carbs – 7.1g, Fat – 15.9g, Protein – 9.95g

69. Tuna Salad

Preparation Time: 18 minutes

Cook time: 0 minutes

Servings: 4

Ingredients:

- 1
- can tuna
- 4 eggs, boiled, peeled and chopped
- 1 oz olives, pitted and sliced
- 1/3 cup cheese cream
- ½ cup almond milk
- ½ tsp ground black pepper
- ½ tsp kosher salt
- 1 tbsp garlic, minced

Directions:

1. In medium bowl, mash tuna with fork.

2. Add chopped eggs and stir.

3. Add sliced olives and stir.

4. In another bowl, whisk together cheese cream and almond milk.

5. Add black pepper, salt and garlic, stir carefully.

6. Add cheese mixture to tuna mixture and mix up.

7. Serve.

Nutrition per Serving: Calories - 182, Carbs - 8g, Fat – 11.9g, Protein - 12.88g

VEGETABLES

70. Broccoli Croquets

Preparation Time: 20 minutes

Cook time: 12 minutes

Servings: 4

Ingredients:

- 10 oz broccoli, chopped roughly
- 1 tsp onion powder
- 1 tsp turmeric
- 1 tsp salt
- 1 tsp paprika
- 3 eggs, beaten
- 1 tbsp flax meal
- 1 cup spinach, chopped into tiny pieces
- ½ cup coconut flour
- 6 oz bacon, chopped
- 4 tbsp butter

Directions:

1. Place broccoli in blender or food processor and blend until smooth.
2. Transfer this mass to bowl and add onion powder, turmeric, salt, and paprika. Stir.
3. Add eggs in bowl and mix until get homogenous mass.
4. Add flax meal and stir.
5. Add spinach to bowl and mix well.
6. Add coconut flour and bacon, stir carefully.
7. Heat up pan on medium heat and melt butter.
8. Shape mixture into croquets 1½-2 inch in diameter and put in

pan.

9. Cook for 4 minutes on both sides.

10. Serve warm.

Nutrition per Serving: Calories - 293, Carbs - 6,45g, Fat – 23.1g, Protein - 15,68g

71. Kale Paste

Preparation Time: 25 minutes

Cook time: 35 minutes

Servings: 4

Ingredients:

- 8 oz spinach, chopped roughly
- 8 oz kale, chopped roughly
- 3 tbsp butter
- ½ cup almond milk
- 1 tsp ground black pepper
- 1 tsp turmeric
- 1 tsp oregano
- 1 tbsp almond flour
- 3 tbsp Parmesan cheese, grated

Directions:

1. Place spinach and kale in blender or food processor and blend for about 3 minutes until get smooth consistency.

2. Heat up pan over medium heat and melt butter.

3. Put vegetable mixture in pan.

4. Pour in almond milk and season with black pepper, oregano and turmeric.

5. Add almond flour and stir gently. Close lid.

6. Simmer dish for 7 minutes.

7. After that, add cheese and stir carefully. Simmer for 3 minutes more.

8. Let dish cool down for few minutes and serve.

Nutrition per Serving: Calories - 271, Carbs – 7.1g, Fat – 24.2g, Protein – 10g

72. Sautéed Broccoli

Preparation Time: 12 minutes

Cook time: 25 minutes

Servings: 3

Ingredients:

- 1 clove garlic

- 5 tbsp olive oil

- 1 lb broccoli florets, steamed

- Salt and ground black pepper to taste

- 1 tbsp Parmesan cheese

Directions:

1. Peel and mince garlic. Grate Parmesan cheese.

2. Preheat pan with oil on medium high heat.

3. Add minced garlic and sauté for 2 minutes.

4. Add steamed broccoli to pan and cook for 15 minutes, stirring occasionally.

5. Season with salt and pepper, stir carefully.

6. Serve topped with Parmesan cheese.

Nutrition per Serving: Calories - 189, Carbs – 5.94g, Fat – 13.85g, Protein – 4.97g

73. Cauliflower in Aromatic Batter

Preparation Time: 12 minutes

Cook time: 23 minutes

Servings: 4

Ingredients:

- 4 eggs, beaten
- ½ cup almond milk
- 1 tsp salt
- 1 tsp ground black pepper
- into medium florets
- ½ cup almond flour
- 1 tsp minced garlic
- 1 tbsp butter
- 14 oz cauliflower, divided

Directions:

1. In bowl, whisk together eggs, almond milk, salt, black pepper, and almond flour.
2. Mix up mixture until smooth.
3. Add garlic and stir.
4. Grease baking dish with butter and put cauliflower florets in it.
5. Pour egg mixture over cauliflower and stir.
6. Set oven to 365 F and heat it up.
7. Place baking dish in oven and bake for 20 minutes.

8.   When time is up, let dish cool down for 3-5 minutes.

9.   Serve hot.

Nutrition per Serving: Calories - 230, Carbs – 8.45g, Fat – 17.9g, Protein - 10g

74. Chopped Cabbage Stew

Preparation Time: 22 minutes

Cook time: 35 minutes

Servings: 8

Ingredients:

- 1 lb beef brisket, cut into 1½ inch cubes
- 1 tbsp kosher salt
- 1 tsp turmeric
- 1 tsp paprika
- 1/3 cup cream
- 2 cups chicken stock
- 2 jalapeno pepper, seeded and chopped
- 4 oz red cabbage, chopped
- 2 lbs white cabbage, chopped
- 5 celery stalks, chopped
- 2 white onions, peeled and sliced

Directions:

1.   Mix beef cubes with salt, turmeric and paprika.
2.   Put meat in saucepan, add cream and chicken stock.
3.   Close lid, heat up saucepan over medium heat and simmer dish for 20 minutes.
4.   Meanwhile, combine jalapeno pepper, cabbage and celery.
5.   Add onion to saucepan, stir and simmer for 5 minutes more.

6. Add cabbage mixture to saucepan, stir and simmer for another 15 minutes on low heat.

7. Let dish cool down for few minutes and serve.

Nutrition per Serving: Calories - 131, Carbs - 6.44g, Fat – 35.9g, Protein - 15.9g

SIDE DISHES

75. Fried Swiss Chard

Preparation Time: 15 minutes

Cook time: 12 minutes

Servings: 3

Ingredients:

- 4 bacon slices
- 1 bunch Swiss chard
- 2 tbsp butter
- 3 tbsp lemon juice
- ½ tsp garlic paste
- Salt and ground black pepper to taste

Directions:

1. Chop bacon slices. Chop Swiss chard.
2. Preheat pan on medium heat. Add chopped bacon and fry until crispy.
3. Toss butter in pan and stir until melts.
4. Add lemon juice and garlic paste, stir. Cook for 1 minute more.
5. Add Swiss chard and stir. Cook for another 4 minutes.
6. Season dish with salt and pepper, stir.
7. Serve hot.

Nutrition per Serving: Calories - 297, Carbs – 5.89g, Fat – 31.8g,

Protein – 7.92g

76. Broccoli Stew

Preparation Time: 12 minutes

Cook time: 25 minutes

Servings: 4

Ingredients:

- 1 cup bok choy, chopped roughly
- 1 cup broccoli, chopped roughly
- 1 tsp kosher salt
- 1 tsp paprika
- ½ quart bone broth
- 5 oz bacon strips
- ½ tsp ground black pepper
- 1 tsp olive oil
- ¼ cup cream cheese
- 1 tbsp cream
- ¼ cup almond milk

Directions:

1. In medium bowl, combine bok choy, broccoli, salt and paprika.
2. Pour bone broth in saucepan.
3. Add vegetable mixture and start to cook on low heat.
4. Season bacon strips with black pepper.
5. Heat up pan with oil over medium heat. Add bacon and cook for 2 minutes.
6. Transfer bacon to saucepan. Stir carefully.
7. In bowl, mix together cream cheese and cream.
8. Add cream mass and almond milk to saucepan. Stir gently.

9. Close lid. Continue simmer stew for 10 minutes.

10. Let stew cool down for few minutes.

11. Serve hot.

Nutrition per Serving: Calories - 211, Carbs - 5g, Fat - 16.84g, Protein - 11.45g

77. Tasty Broccoli Mash

Preparation Time: 12 minutes

Cook time: 18 minutes

Servings: 4

Ingredients:

- 1 cup water
- 14 oz broccoli, chopped roughly
- 1 tsp kosher salt
- ¼ cup coconut milk
- 2 tbsp butter
- 3 oz Parmesan cheese, grated
- 1 oz olives, pitted and sliced

Directions:

1. Pour water in saucepan. Add broccoli and ½ teaspoon salt.

2. Cover and cook broccoli for 10 minutes on medium heat.

3. In medium bowl, whisk together coconut milk, butter and ½ teaspoon salt.

4. When broccoli is cooked, place it in blender or food processor and blend until smooth.

5. Add butter mixture in broccoli and stir.

6. Add cheese and olives in broccoli mixture.

7. Mix up until get homogenous consistency.

8. Serve.

Nutrition per Serving: Calories - 128, Carbs - 5.85g, Fat - 11g, Protein - 6.9g

78. Twice-Baked Zucchini

Preparation Time: 12 minutes

Cook time: 35 minutes

Servings: 4

Ingredients:

- 2 zucchini
- 2 tbsp butter
- 1 tbsp jalapeño pepper, seeded and chopped
- 2 oz onion, peeled and chopped
- 4 bacon strips, cooked and crumbled
- 2 oz cream cheese, softened
- 4 oz cheddar cheese, shredded
- ¼ cup sour cream
- Salt and ground black pepper to taste

Directions:

1. Cut zucchini into half and each half in half lengthwise.

2. Scoop out flesh and put in bowl. Place zucchini cups in

baking dish.

3. In mixing bowl, combine zucchini flesh, butter, jalapeño pepper, onion, bacon, cream cheese, cheddar cheese, sour cream, salt and pepper. Mix well.

4. Set oven to 350 F and heat it up.

5. Spread this mixture in zucchini quarters and place baking dish in oven.

6. Bake for 30 minutes. Serve.

Nutrition per Serving: Calories - 258, Carbs – 2.98g, Fat – 21.9g, Protein – 9.9g

79. Zucchini Wraps with the Cream Cheese

Preparation Time: 15 minutes

Cook time: 5 minutes

Servings: 4

Ingredients:

- 1 zucchini, washed and sliced
- 1 tsp paprika
- ½ tsp ground black pepper
- 2 tbsp coconut oil
- 1/3 cup cream cheese
- 1 tbsp minced garlic
- 7 oz Parmesan cheese, grated

Directions:

1. In bowl, mix together zucchini, paprika and black pepper.

2. Heat up pan with coconut oil over medium heat.

3. Fry zucchini for 30 seconds on each side.

4. Transfer zucchini slices to paper towels and drain grease.

5. In bowl, combine garlic with cream cheese. Mix up until get homogenous mass.

6. Add Parmesan cheese and stir carefully.

7. Grease zucchini slices with cream cheese mixture and wrap rolls.

8. Serve.

Nutrition per Serving: Calories - 301, Carbs – 4.98g, Fat - 25g, Protein – 17.9g

80. Cheddar and Ham Wraps

Preparation Time: 10 minutes

Cook time: 7 minutes

Servings: 1

Ingredients:

- 2 tbsp mayonnaise

- 1 low carb wrap

- 2 oz cheddar, shredded

- 2 oz deli ham, slices

- Pickles or jalapenos to taste, sliced

- Salt and ground black pepper to taste

Directions:

1. Spread mayonnaise on low carb wrap.

2. Sprinkle with shredded cheese.

3. Add ham slices.

4. Add jalapenos or pickles to taste.

5. Sprinkle with salt and black pepper to tasty.

6. Wrap it up and serve.

Nutrition per Serving: Calories - 595, Carbs – 7.9g, Fat – 43.7g, Protein – 26.8g

81. Easy Avocado Wraps

Preparation Time: 10 minutes

Cook time: 0 minutes

Servings: 1

Ingredients:

- 3 lettuce leaves
- 3 tbsp mayonnaise
- 6 strips bacon, cooked
- ½ roma tomato, sliced
- ½ avocado, sliced
- Salt and ground black pepper to taste

Directions:

1. Carefully flatten lettuce leaves and add tablespoon of mayonnaise to each.

2. Then put 2 bacon strips on each leaf.

3. Then place tomato and avocado on top.

4. Sprinkle with salt and black pepper.

5. Wrap each leaf tightly. Serve.

Nutrition per Serving: Calories - 633, Carbs – 5.9g, Fat – 55.5g, Protein – 17.8g

82. Crispy Zucchini Circles with Parmesan Cheese

Preparation Time: 25 minutes

Cook time: 33 minutes

Servings: 4

Ingredients:

- 2 zucchini, washed and sliced
- 1 tsp basil
- ½ tsp cilantro
- 7 oz Cheddar cheese, grated
- 6 oz Parmesan cheese, grated
- 1 tbsp butter
- ½ tbsp minced garlic
- 1 tbsp coconut oil

Directions:

1. In medium bowl, combine zucchini slices, basil and cilantro.
2. In another bowl, mix together Cheddar cheese, Parmesan cheese, garlic and butter.
3. Set oven to 370 F and heat it up.

4. Cover the tray with the baking paper and transfer the sliced zucchini in the tray.

5. Season zucchini slices with cheese mixture and spray with coconut oil.

6. Place tray in oven and bake for 15 minutes.

7. Let dish cool down for 4-6 minutes and serve.

Nutrition per Serving: Calories - 269, Carbs - 4g, Fat – 20.9g, Protein - 18.45g

83. Baked Cauliflower Casserole

Preparation Time: 15 minutes

Cook time: 35 minutes

Servings: 4

Ingredients:

- 10 oz cauliflower, divided into small florets
- ½ tsp salt
- 1 tsp ground black pepper
- 4 eggs, beaten
- 1/3 cup coconut milk
- 2 tsp butter
- 5 oz green beans
- 7 oz Parmesan cheese, grated

Directions:

1. In bowl, combine cauliflower florets with salt and black pepper.

2. In another bowl, whisk together eggs and coconut milk.

3. Grease baking form with butter and put cauliflower florets in it.

4. Place green beans on top.

5. Pour egg mixture over green beans and sprinkle with cheese.

6. Set oven to 365 F and heat it up.

7. Place dish in oven and bake for 30 minutes.

8. Let it cool briefly and serve it immediately.

Nutrition per Serving: Calories - 309, Carbs - 10g, Fat – 20.9g, Protein – 23.9g

84. Spicy Roasted Asparagus

Preparation Time: 15 minutes

Cook time: 17 minutes

Servings: 4

Ingredients:

- 10 oz asparagus, washed and chopped roughly
- 1 tsp salt
- 2 tsp thyme
- 1 tsp minced garlic
- 1 tsp oregano
- 4 tbsp butter
- 1 tbsp lemon juice
- 1 oz walnuts, crushed
- ½ cup chicken stock

Directions:

1. In medium bowl, combine asparagus, salt, thyme, garlic, and oregano.

2. Preheat pan on medium high heat and melt butter.

3. Add lemon juice and bring liquid to boil.

4. Add crushed walnuts, stir.

5. Add asparagus and pour chicken stock. Stir well.

6. Close lid and simmer for 10 minutes on medium heat, until asparagus is soft.

7. Remove excess liquid from pan and serve dish.

Nutrition per Serving: Calories - 129, Carbs - 3.68g, Fat - 13g, Protein - 3g

FAT BOMBS

85. Absolute Cacao Fat Bombs

Serves: 8

Preparation Time:10 minutes

Ingredients

- 1/2 cup of coconut oil, melted
- 3/4 cup heavy cream
- 1/4 cup cacao dry powder, unsweetened
- 3 Tbsp of almond butter
- 1 tsp nutmeg (optional)
- 4 drops of natural sweeter stevia, or to taste

Directions

1. Melt the coconut oil in a microwave for 10 - 15 seconds.
2. Combine all ingredients in a bowl and stir well.
3. Pour the mixture in a cake moulds and freeze for two hours or until set.
4. Press out of molds and place on a plate or in a container.
5. Keep refrigerated.

Nutrition per Serving: Calories: 239 Carbohydrates: 3.5g Proteins: 3g Fat: 26g Fiber: 2g

86. Zucchini Fat Bomb

Serves: 8

Preparation Time:15 minutes

Ingredients

- 2 Tbsp almond butter
- 3 large zucchini shredded
- 1 cup fresh basil and chives finely chopped
- 1 cup shredded mozzarella
- 1/2 cup Cheddar cheese
- Pinch of salt (optional)

Directions

1. Peel zucchini, and shred in a food processor.
2. Line one baking sheet with parchment paper.
3. In a mixing bowl, combine all ingredients in a compact mixture.
4. For mixture into small balls, and place them on a prepared baking sheet.
5. Freeze for 2 - 3 hours in a freezer.
6. Serve. Keep refrigerated.

Nutrition per Serving: Calories: 108 Carbohydrates: 3g Proteins: 8g Fat: 8g Fiber: 1g

87. Almonds Gale Fat Bombs

Serves: 12

Preparation Time:10 minutes

Ingredients

- 1 cup coconut oil
- 1 cup almond butter (plain, unsalted)
- 1/4 cup ground almonds (without salt)
- 1 tsp vanilla extract
- 1/4 can natural sweetener such Stevia, Erythritol, Truvia,...etc.
- Pinch of salt

Directions

1. In a microwave safe bowl, softened the coconut butter.
2. Add all ingredients in your fast-speed blender.
3. Blend until thoroughly combined.
4. Make small balls and place on a plate lined with parchment paper.
5. Freeze for about 4 hours or overnight.
6. Serve.

Nutrition per Serving: Calories: 301 Carbohydrates: 5g Proteins: 6g Fat: 30g Fiber: 2g

88. Bacon and Basil Fat Bombs

Serves: 8

Preparation Time:15 minutes

Ingredients

- 2 cups of cream cheese from refrigerator
- 6 slices of bacon, finely chopped
- 1 small chili pepper, finely chopped
- 1 Tbsp fresh basil (chopped)
- 1/2 tsp onion powder
- 1/4 tsp garlic powder
- Salt and pepper to taste

Directions

1. Beat the cheese cream in a mixing bowl.
2. Add chopped bacon and stir well with the spoon.
3. Add all remaining ingredients and stir well to combine all ingredients.
4. Make small balls and place on a platter.
5. Refrigerate for 2 - 3 hours and serve.
6. Keep refrigerated.

Nutrition per Serving: Calories: 265 Carbohydrates: 2g Proteins: 6g Fat: 27g Fiber: 0.03g

89. Berries and Maca Fat Bombs

Serves: 8

Preparation Time:15 minutes

Ingredients

- 2 cups fresh cream

- 2 Tbsp fresh butter, softened

- 1/2 cup of natural granulated sweetener (Stevia, Erythritol...etc.)

- 1/2 cup frozen berries thawed (blueberries, bilberries, raspberries)

- 2 tsp Maca root powder

- 1 Tbsp arrowroot powder (or chia seeds as thickener)

- 1 tsp vanilla extract

Directions

1. Beat the cream with a hand mixer in a bowl until double in volume and stiff.
2. Add all remaining ingredients and continue to beat until combined completely.
3. Pour the berries mixture in ice cubes tray or in a muffin tray.
4. Freeze for at least 4 hours (preferably overnight).
5. Serve or Keep refrigerated.

Nutrition per Serving: Calories: 152 Carbohydrates: 6g Proteins: 2g Fat: 15g Fiber: 0.5g

90. Chilly Tuna Fat Balls

Serves: 8

Preparation Time:10 minutes

Ingredients

- 2 cans tuna, drained
- 1 medium avocado, cubed
- 2 Tbsp coconut butter
- 1/2 cup mayonnaise
- 2 Tbsp mustard
- 1 cup Parmesan cheese
- 1/3 cup ground almonds
- 1 tsp garlic powder
- Salt and pepper to taste

Directions

1. Cut medium avocado in half, remove the pit and skin, and cut the flesh in cubes.
2. Drain and add tuna in a large bawl along with all ingredients; stir well with the spoon.
3. Make the tuna mixture into small bowls
4. Place tuna balls on a plate lined with parchment paper, and refrigerate for 2 hours.
5. Serve or keep refrigerated.

Nutrition per Serving: Calories: 197 Carbohydrates: 6g Proteins: 9g Fat: 17g Fiber: 2.2g

91. Choco - Peanut Butter Fat Balls

Serves: 12

Preparation Time:15 minutes

Ingredients

- 1/2 cup fresh cream
- 1 cup of dark chocolate chips (60 - 69& cacao solid)
- 1/2 cup of peanut butter, softened
- 1/4 cup of coconut oil, softened
- 1/4 cup of fresh butter, softened
- 2 Tbsp ground peanuts

Directions

1. In a bowl, beat the cream until stiff peak and double in volume.
2. Melt the chocolate chips in a microwave for about 45 - 60 seconds; stir every 20 seconds.
3. Fold all ingredients in a whipped cream and beat for 2 - 3 minutes.
4. In a meanwhile, whip together peanut butter, coconut oil and butter.
5. Pour the mixture in molds or in cupcakes holders and freeze for 4 hours.
6. Keep refrigerated.

Nutrition per Serving: Calories: 310 Carbohydrates: 7g Proteins: 5g Fat: 28g Fiber: 2g

92. Cinnamon - Nutmeg Fat Bombs

Serves: 8

Preparation Time:10 minutes

Ingredients

- 1 cup almond butter (plain, unsalted)
- 1/2 cup almond milk (or coconut milk)
- 3/4 cup ground almonds or Macadamia nuts (unsalted)
- 1/2 tsp cinnamon
- 1 tsp vanilla extract
- 1/2 tsp ground nutmeg (optional)
- 2 Tbsp of natural sweetener (Stevia, Truvia, Erythritol...etc.)

Directions

1. Add all ingredients in your food processor, and process for 45 - 60 seconds.
2. Add more or less sweetener, to taste.
3. Grease your hands with oil and form dough into small balls.
4. Place on a baking pan covered with parchment paper and refrigerate for 2 - 3 hours.
5. Serve.

Nutrition per Serving: Calories: 274 Carbohydrates: 6.5g Proteins: 11g Fat: 24g Fiber: 3.5g

93. Creamy Green Olives Fat Bombs

Serves: 8

Preparation Time:20 minutes

Ingredients

- 1 lb cold cream cheese
- 1 cup whipped cream
- 1 1/2 cups green olives pitted
- 1/2 cup fresh parsley finely chopped
- 1 pinch of salt (optional)

Directions

1. Line a platter or baking pan with parchment paper; set aside.
2. Add cream cheese in a bowl and fast whisk with the spoon.
3. In a separate bowl, beat the cream to double in volume.
4. Combine the cream cheese and whipped cream; season with a pinch of salt.
5. Make balls from the cream cheese mixture, and insert one olive in a centre of each ball.
6. Roll each ball in chopped parsley and coat evenly from all sides.
7. Place the balls on prepared platter and refrigerate for 4 hours or overnight
8. Serve.

Nutrition per Serving: Calories: 131 Carbohydrates: 2g Proteins: 2g Fat: 14g Fiber: 0.5g

94. Creamy Lime Fat Bombs

Serves: 10

Preparation Time:10 minutes

Ingredients

- 3/4 cup coconut oil
- 1/2 cup fresh cream (yields 2 cups whipped)
- 1/2 cup cream cheese
- 1 tsp pure lime extract
- 10 drops natural sweetener (Stevia, Truvia, Erythritol...etc.)

Directions

1. In a bowl, beat the cream with a hand mixer.
2. Add all remaining ingredients and continue to beat for 45 - 60 seconds.
3. Pour the mixture into a silicone tray and freeze for several hours.
4. When hard enough, remove from the freezer, and from silicone tray and serve.

Nutrition per Serving: Calories: 223 Carbohydrates: 1g Proteins: 1g Fat: 25g Fiber: 0g

95. Eggs with Gorgonzola Fat Bombs

Serves: 6

Preparation Time:10 minutes

Ingredients

- 2 eggs, boiled
- 1/4 cup fresh butter, softened
- 1 cup cream cheese full-fat
- 3/4 cup Gorgonzola - blue cheese, grated

Directions

1. First, boil the eggs in a saucepan; remove from heat and set aside for 10 minutes.
2. In a meantime, line a baking pan with parchment paper.
3. Combine cream cheese, butter and grated Gorgonzola. Add the chopped eggs and stir well.
4. Make 6 - 8 balls and place them on a prepared pan.
5. Refrigerate for 2 - 3 hours and serve.

Nutrition per Serving: Calories: 274 Carbohydrates: 2g Proteins: 8g Fat: 27g Fiber: 0g

96. Lemon Lilliputian Fat Bombs

Serves: 10

Preparation Time:10 minutes

Ingredients

- 1/2 cup coconut oil, melted and cooled
- 1/4 cup heavy cream
- 1/4 cup cream cheese, full-fat
- 1 lemon, freshly squeezed
- 1 lemon zest (finely grated fresh)

- 1 tsp pure lemon extract

- 1/4 cup natural sweetener (Stevia, Erythritol...etc.)

- 1/2 cup coconut shredded, unsweetened

Directions

1. Melt the coconut oil in a microwave oven for 10 - 15 seconds. Set aside to cool for 2 to 3 minutes.

2. Whisk melted coconut oil with heavy cream, and with the cream cheese.

3. Pour the lemon juice and lemon zest and stir. Add stevia sweetener and stir well until sweetener dissolve completely..

4. At the end, add pure lemon extract and stir.

5. Pour the mixture in a candy molds or ice cube tray.

6. Freeze for two hours, and then remove your fat bombs on a platter.

7. Keep refrigerated.

Nutrition per Serving: Calories: 165 Carbohydrates: .5g Proteins: 1g Fat: 17g Fiber: 1g

SNACKS

97. Chicken Wings with Tomato Dip

Preparation Time:50 minutes

Servings:6

Nutritional value per serving: 236 Calories; 13.5g Fat; 6g Carbs;
19.4g Protein; 2.8g Sugars

Ingredients

- 12 chicken wings

- Salt and pepper, to taste

- For the Tomato Dip:

- 4 ripe tomatoes, crushed

- 1 onion, finely chopped

- 1 cup mango, peeled and chopped

- 1 teaspoon chili pepper, deveined and finely minced

- 2 heaping tablespoons cilantro, finely chopped

- 2 tablespoons lime juice

Directions

1. Start by preheating your oven to 400 degrees F. Set a wire
   rack inside a rimmed baking sheet.

2. Season chicken wings with salt and pepper. Bake wings
   approximately 45 minutes or until skin is crispy.

3. Then, thoroughly combine all ingredients for the tomato dip.
   Place in your refrigerator until ready to serve.

98. Spicy Tuna Deviled Eggs

Preparation Time:20 minutes

Servings:6

Nutritional value per serving: 203 Calories; 13.3g Fat; 3.8g Carbs; 17.2g Protein; 1.5g Sugars

Ingredients

- 12 eggs

- 1/3 cup mayonnaise

- 1 can tuna in spring water, drained

- 1/2 teaspoon smoked cayenne pepper

- 1/4 teaspoon fresh or dried dill weed

- 2 pickled jalapenos, minced

- Salt and black pepper, to taste

Directions

1. Place the eggs in a wide pot; cover with cold water by 1 inch. Bring to a rapid boil.

2. Decrease the heat to medium-low; let them simmer an additional 10 minutes.

3. Peel the eggs and rinse them under running water.

4. Slice each egg in half lengthwise and remove the yolks. Thoroughly combine the yolks with the remaining ingredients.

5. Divide the mixture among egg whites and arrange deviled eggs on a nice serving platter. Enjoy!

99. Broccoli and Goat Cheese Dip

Preparation Time:10 minutes

Servings:8

Nutritional value per serving: 134 Calories; 10.2g Fat; 6.5g Carbs; 5.1g Protein; 1.7g Sugars

Ingredients

- 1 pound broccoli, broken into florets
- 1/2 cup sour cream
- 1/2 cup goat cheese
- 1 teaspoon shallot powder
- 1 teaspoon Italian seasoning mix
- 1 teaspoon garlic powder
- 1/3 cup mayonnaise

Directions

1. Steam the broccoli for 4 to 5 minutes or until crisp-tender. Transfer to a food processor.

2. Add the remaining ingredients, except for mayonnaise. Puree in the food processor until well blended.

3. Stir in mayonnaise and puree until creamy, uniform and smooth. Serve well-chilled and enjoy!

100. Cheese, Mortadella and Salami Roll-Ups

Preparation Time:10 minutes

Servings:5

Nutritional value per serving: 381 Calories; 31.2g Fat; 4.8g Carbs; 17.6g Protein; 1.7g Sugars

Ingredients

- 10 slices Provolone cheese
- 4 ounces mayonnaise
- 10 slices Mortadella
- 10 slices Genoa salami
- 10 olives, pitted

Directions

1. Spread a thin layer of mayo onto each slice of cheese. Add a slice of Mortadella on top of the mayo.
2. Top with a slice of Genoa salami. Roll them up; place olives on the top and secure with toothpicks.
3. Serve immediately.

101. Paprika and Mustard Bacon Chips

Preparation Time:20 minutes

Servings:4

Nutritional value per serving: 118 Calories; 10g Fat; 1.9g Carbs;

5g Protein; 0.4g Sugars

Ingredients

- 12 bacon strips, cut into small squares

- 1 tablespoon smoked paprika

- 1 tablespoon mustard

Directions

1. Preheat your oven to 360 degrees F

2. Toss the bacon strips with paprika and mustard.

3. Arrange bacon squares on a parchment lined baking sheet. Bake for 10 to 15 minutes. Enjoy!

102. Easy Rutabaga Fries

Preparation Time:35 minutes

Servings:4

Nutritional value per serving: 134 Calories; 10.8g Fat; 5.9g Carbs; 1.5g Protein; 3.8g Sugars

Ingredients

- 1 ½ pounds rutabaga, cut into sticks 1/4-inch wide

- 3 tablespoons olive oil

- Salt and ground black pepper, to taste

- 1/2 teaspoon cayenne pepper

- 1/2 teaspoon mustard seeds

Directions

1. Add rutabaga sticks to a mixing dish. In another small-sized mixing dish, whisk the other ingredients.

2. Add the oil mixture to the rutabaga sticks and toss to coat well.

3. Preheat your oven to 440 degrees F. Line a baking sheet with parchment paper.

4. Place seasoned rutabaga sticks on the baking sheet. Roast them approximately 30 minutes, turning baking sheet occasionally. Serve warm and enjoy!

103. Dilled Chicken Wingettes with Goat Cheese Dip

Preparation Time:1 hour 15 minutes

Servings:10

Nutritional value per serving: 227 Calories; 10.2g Fat; 0.4g Carbs; 31.5g Protein; 0.2g Sugars

Ingredients

- Nonstick cooking spray
- 3 pounds chicken wingettes
- Salt and black pepper, to taste
- 1/4 teaspoon smoked paprika
- 1 teaspoon dried dill weed

For Goat Cheese Dip:

- 1 cup goat cheese, crumbled
- 1/3 cup mayonnaise
- 2 tablespoons Greek-style yogurt

- 1 teaspoon Dijon mustard

- 2 cloves garlic, smashed

- 1 teaspoon onion powder

- 1/2 teaspoon ground cumin

- 1/4 cup fresh coriander leaves, finely chopped

Directions

1. Preheat your oven to 390 degrees F. Set a wire rack inside a rimmed baking sheet. Spritz the rack with a nonstick cooking oil.

2. Toss chicken wingettes with salt, pepper, paprika, and dill.

3. Place the chicken wingettes skin side up on the rack. Bake in the lower quarter of the oven for 30 to 35 minutes.

4. Turn the oven up to 420 degrees F. Bake for a further 40 minutes on the higher shelf, rotating the baking sheet once.

5. In the meantime, combine goat cheese, mayo, yogurt, mustard, garlic, onion powder and ground cumin. Serve with warm wingettes, garnished with fresh cilantro.

104. Cheese, Ham and Greek Yogurt Dip

Preparation Time:5 minutes

Servings:6

Nutritional value per serving: 147 Calories; 10.6g Fat; 2.7g Carbs; 10.2g Protein; 0.2g Sugars

Ingredients

- 5 ounces Greek yogurt

- 5 ounces Ricotta cheese, at room temperature

- 1 cup Colby cheese, shredded

- 1/2 cup ham, crumbled

- 2 tablespoons fresh parsley, chopped

Directions

1. Thoroughly combine all of the above ingredients, except for parsley, in a mixing dish.

2. Garnish with fresh parsley. Serve with veggie sticks. Bon appétit!

105. Cocktail Salad on a Stick

Preparation Time:10 minutes

Servings:6

Nutritional value per serving: 249 Calories; 19.3g Fat; 6g Carbs; 9.7g Protein; 2.1g Sugars

Ingredients

- 2 cans of tiny pickled beets, drained and rinsed

- 2 bell peppers, sliced

- 4 ounces blue cheese, cubed

- 1 cup prosciutto, sliced

- 1/2 cup olives, pitted

- 1/3 cup champagne vinegar

- 1/3 cup olive oil

- 1/2 teaspoon cumin seeds

Directions

1. Tread pickled beets, bell peppers, blue cheese, prosciutto, and olives onto cocktail sticks.

2. Drizzle with champagne vinegar and olive oil; sprinkle with cumin seeds. Bon appétit!

106. Greek-Style Meat and Cheese Dip

Preparation Time:10 minutes

Servings:24

Nutritional value per serving: 153 Calories; 11.2g Fat; 2.2g Carbs; 10.8g Protein; 0.6g Sugars

Ingredients

- 1 pound ground beef
- 1/2 pound ground lamb
- 2 cups sour cream
- 1 cup cream cheese
- 1 cup feta cheese
- 1/2 cup tomato puree
- 2 garlic cloves, minced
- 1 sprig dried rosemary, crushed
- 1 sprig dried thyme, crushed
- 1 cup Kalamata olives, pitted and sliced

Directions

1. Brown ground meat in a pan that is preheated over a medium-high heat. Crumble with a wide spatula and set aside.

2. In a large bowl, thoroughly combine the remaining ingredients, except for olives.

3. Layer the cheese mixture with meat mixture. Top with sliced Kalamata olives and serve with your favorite dippers.

107. Celery Root French Fries with Pine Nuts

Preparation Time:35 minutes

Servings:6

Nutritional value per serving: 96 Calories; 8.5g Fat; 4.1g Carbs; 1.5g Protein; 1.7g Sugars

Ingredients

- 1 ½ pounds celery root, cut into sticks
- Salt and ground black pepper, to taste
- 1/2 teaspoon cayenne pepper
- 2 tablespoons olive oil
- 1 tablespoon Cajun seasoning
- 1/4 cup pine nuts, coarsely ground

Directions

1. Preheat your oven to 390 degrees F. Line a baking sheet with a parchment paper or Silpat mat.
2. Mix celery root, salt, black pepper, cayenne pepper, olive oil and Cajun seasoning in a mixing dish.
3. Arrange celery stick on the prepared baking sheet and bake for 30 minutes, flipping every 10 minutes to promote even cooking.
4. Arrange on a serving platter and sprinkle with pine nuts. Serve hot with a homemade mayo or seafood dipping sauce. Bon appétit!

108. Egg Free Roasted Herb Crackers

Preparation Time: 20 minutes

Cook Time: 120 minutes

Servings: 15

Ingredients

- 10 celery sticks

- 3 cups of roughly ground flax seed

- 2 tbsps. of raw apple cider vinegar

- ¼ cup avocado oil

- 1 tsp. Himalayan rock salt

- about 0.2 oz. fresh rosemary leaves

- about 0.2 oz. fresh thyme leaves

Directions

1. Preheat your oven to 225°F.

2. Cover two large baking sheets with parchment paper then set aside.

3. Place salt, herbs, celery, oil, and vinegar in the bowl of your food processor and pulse until the celery is properly pureed.

4. Add ground flax and pulse again until it's well-combined.

5. Allow it to sit 2 minutes to firm up.

6. Plop half the dough onto your prepared baking sheet and, with the back of your spoon, smoothen it out until it covers the entire baking sheet. The crackers should be about ¼-inch thick.

7. As soon as it is completed, repeat with the remaining dough on the other baking sheet and run a knife along the sheets, scoring squares in the dough.

8. Bake 2 hours and, halfway through baking, remove the

parchment paper and flip the crackers. Note the baking time will greatly vary depending on the thickness of the crackers. You want the result to be crunchy and crisp without moisture.

9. Remove from the oven and leave it to cool on the baking sheet about 15 minutes.

Nutritional value per serving:

- Calories: 158
- Fat: 10.8g
- Carbohydrates: 7.7g
- Protein: 4.4g
- Sugar: 0.7g

109. Pork Rind Puppy Chow

Preparation Time: 1 hour

Servings: 8

Ingredients

- oz. (4 cups) pork rinds
- ⅛ tsp. vanilla extract
- ¼ cup of coconut oil
- 12 drops of liquid stevia
- 4 tbsps. of butter
- 3 tbsps. unsweetened cocoa powder
- ½ cup all-natural peanut butter

Directions

1. Melt the peanut butter, coconut oil, and butter in a small saucepan or microwave.

2. Mix in the vanilla, cocoa powder, and stevia.

3. Pour pork rinds into the freezer bag and pour chocolate over pork rinds.

4. Seal the bag and toss to coat.

5. Keep in the fridge and allow it to cool 30-60 minutes. Enjoy!

Nutritional value per serving:

-   Calories: 285

-   Fat: 25g

-   Carbohydrates: 4g

-   Protein: 12g

-   Sugars: 1g

DESSERTS

110. Cheesy Coconut Cake

Preparation Time:30 minutes

Servings:12

Nutritional value per serving: 246 Calories; 22.2g Fat; 6.7g Carbs; 8.1g Protein; 1.9g Sugars

Ingredients

- 10 ounces almond meal
- 1 ounce coconut, shredded
- 1 teaspoon baking powder
- 1/8 teaspoon salt
- 4 eggs, lightly beaten
- 3 ounces stevia
- 1/2 stick butter
- 5 ounces coconut yogurt
- 5 ounces cream cheese

Directions

1. Start by preheating your oven to 350 degrees F. Spritz 2 spring form pans with a nonstick cooking spray.

2. In a mixing bowl, thoroughly combine the almond meal, coconut and baking powder. Stir in the salt, eggs and 2 ounces of stevia.

3. Combine the 2 mixtures and stir until everything is well incorporated.

4. Transfer the mixture into 2 spring form pans, introduce in the oven at 350 degrees F; bake for 20 to 25 minutes.

5. Transfer to a wire rack to cool completely. In the meantime, mix the other ingredients, including the remaining 1 ounce of stevia.

6. Place one cake layer on a plate; spread half of the cream cheese filling over it. Now, top with another cake layer; spread the rest of the cream cheese filling over the top. Bon appétit!

111. Coconut Apple Cobbler

Preparation Time:30 minutes

Servings:8

Nutritional value per serving: 152 Calories; 11.8g Fat; 6.7g Carbs; 2.5g Protein;4.4g Sugars

Ingredients

- 2 ½ cups apples, cored and sliced
- 1/2 tablespoon fresh lemon juice
- 1/3 teaspoon xanthan gum
- 1 cup almond flour
- , melted
- 1/4 cup coconut flour
- 3/4 cup xylitol
- 2 eggs, whisked
- 5 tablespoons coconut oil

Directions

1. Start by preheating your oven to 360 degrees F. Lightly grease a baking dish with a nonstick cooking spray.

2. Arrange the apples on the bottom of the baking dish. Drizzle with lemon juice and xanthan gum.

3. Then, in a mixing bowl, mix the flour with xylitol and eggs until the mixture resembles coarse meal. Spread this mixture over the apples.

4. Drizzle coconut oil over topping. Bake for 25 minutes or until dough rises. Bon appétit!

112. Summer Frappe Dessert

Preparation Time: 2 hours

Servings: 2

Nutritional value per serving: 371 Calories; 37.8g Fat; 7.1g Carbs; 3.4g Protein; 4.1g Sugars

Ingredients

- 2 teaspoons instant coffee
- 4 drops liquid Stevia
- 1 tablespoon cacao butter
- 1/4 cup cold water
- 16 raspberries, frozen
- 1 cup almond milk
- 2 tablespoons coconut whipped cream

Directions

1. Combine instant coffee, Stevia, cacao butter and cold water. Shake with a drink mixer for 20 seconds.

2. Place frozen raspberries in dessert glasses. Pour the coffee mixture over it. Add almond milk and ice cubes, if desired.

3. Now, freeze for at least 2 hours or until firm. Serve topped with coconut whipped cream. Enjoy!

113. Cheesecake Cupcakes with Vanilla Frosting

Preparation Time: 30 minutes + chilling time

Servings:8

Nutritional value per serving: 165 Calories; 15.6g Fat; 5.4g Carbs; 5.2g Protein; 0.2g Sugars

Ingredients

For the Muffins:

- 3 tablespoons coconut oil
- 10 ounces Ricotta cheese, at room temperature
- 1 tablespoon rum
- 2 eggs
- freshly grated

- 2 packets stevia
- 1/8 teaspoon ground cloves
- 1/4 teaspoon ground cinnamon
- 1/8 teaspoon nutmeg, preferably

For the Frosting:

- 1/2 cup confectioners' Swerve
- 1/2 stick butter, softened
- 1 teaspoon vanilla
- 1 ½ tablespoons full-fat milk

Directions

1. Preheat your oven to 360 degrees F; coat muffin cups with cupcake liners.
2. Thoroughly combine coconut oil, Ricotta cheese, rum, eggs, stevia, cloves, cinnamon and nutmeg in your food processor.
3. Scrape the batter into the muffin tin; bake for 13 to 16 minutes. Now, place in the freezer for 2 hours.

4. In the meantime, combine confectioners' Swerve with butter and vanilla with an electric mixer.

5. Slowly pour in milk in order to make a spreadable mixture. Frosts chilled cheesecake cupcakes. Bon appétit!

114. Easy Almond Fudge

Preparation Time:3 hours

Servings:8

Nutritional value per serving: 180 Calories; 18.3g Fat; 4.5g Carbs; 1g Protein; 0.5g Sugars

Ingredients

- 3/4 cup almond butter, sugar-free, preferably homemade
- 1 stick butter
- 1/3 cup coconut milk
- 1/4 cup xylitol
- 1/8 teaspoon salt
- 1/8 teaspoon grated nutmeg
- 3 tablespoons xylitol
- 3 tablespoons butter, melted
- 1 teaspoon vanilla essence
- 3 tablespoons cocoa powder

Directions

1. Microwave almond butter and regular butter until they melt.

2. Add coconut milk, 1/4 cup xylitol, salt, and nutmeg; stir to combine well and press into a well-greased glass baking dish.

3. Refrigerate for 2 to 3 hours or until set.

4. In a mixing bowl, make the sauce by whisking 3 tablespoons xylitol, 3 tablespoons of butter melted, vanilla essence and

cocoa powder.

5. Spread the sauce over your fudge. Cut into squares and store in an airtight container.

115. Peanut Ice Cream

Preparation Time:10 minutes + chilling time

Servings:4

Nutritional value per serving: 305 Calories; 18.3g Fat; 4.5g Carbs; 1g Protein; 0.5g Sugars

Ingredients

- 1 ¼ cups almond milk
- 1/3 cup whipped cream
- 17 drops liquid stevia
- 1/2 cup peanuts, chopped
- 1/2 teaspoon xanthan gum

Directions

1. Combine all of the above ingredients, except for xanthan gum, with an electric mixer.

2. Now, stir in xanthan gum, whisking constantly, until the mixture is thick.

3. Then, prepare your ice cream in a machine following manufacturer's instructions.

4. Serve directly from the machine or store in your freezer.

116. Coconut Chia Pudding

Preparation Time:30 minutes

Servings:4

Nutritional value per serving: 270 Calories; 24.7g Fat; 6.5g Carbs; 4.6g Protein; 2.1g Sugars

Ingredients

- 1/3 cup chia seeds
- 1/2 cup water
- 1 cup coconut cream
- 1/2 cup sour cream
- 1/3 teaspoon vanilla extract
- 1 teaspoon key lime zest
- 1/4 teaspoon ground cinnamon
- 2 tablespoons granular Swerve

Directions

1. In a bowl, place all ingredients and stir well; let it sit at least 30 minutes.
2. Divide among individual bowls to serve.
3. Can be stored in the refrigerator up to 3 days.

117. Festive Cake with Cream Cheese Frosting

Preparation Time:40 minutes + chilling time

Servings:10

Nutritional value per serving: 241 Calories; 22.6g Fat; 4.2g Carbs; 6.6g Protein; 2.9g Sugars

Ingredients

- 2/3 cup coconut flour
- 1 ½ cups almond flour
- 1/2 teaspoon baking soda

- 1/2 teaspoon baking powder
- A pinch of salt
- A pinch of grated nutmeg
- 1/2 teaspoon Konjac root fiber
- 1 cup Swerve teaspoon
- fresh ginger, grated
- 2 ½ tablespoons ghee
- 4 eggs
- 1 cup coconut milk, sugar-free
- 1 teaspoon rum extract
- 1 teaspoon vanilla extract

For the Cream Cheese Frosting:

- 10 ounces cream cheese, cold
- 1/3 cup powdered granular sweetener
- 3 ounces butter, at room temperature
- 1 teaspoon vanilla
- A few drops chocolate flavor

Directions

1. Start by preheating your oven to 360 degrees F. Line a baking pan with parchment paper.

2. In a mixing bowl, combine coconut flour, almond flour, baking soda, baking powder, salt, nutmeg, Konjac root fiber, Swerve, and ginger.

3. Microwave ghee until melted and add to the dry mixture in the mixing bowl. Fold in the eggs, one at a time, and stir until combined.

4. Lastly, pour in coconut milk, rum extract, and vanilla extract until your batter is light and fluffy.

5. Press the mixture into the prepared baking pan. Bake for 28 to 33 minutes or until a cake tester inserted in center comes out clean and dry.

6. Let it cool to room temperature.

7. Meanwhile, beat the cream cheese with an electric mixer until

smooth. Stir in powdered granular sweetener and beat again. Beat in the vanilla until it is completely incorporated.

8. Add the butter, vanilla, and chocolate flavor; whip until light, fluffy and uniform. Frost the cake and serve well-chilled. Bon appétit!

118. Sinfully Delicious Whiskey Chocolate Bites

Preparation Time:10 minutes + chilling time

Servings:8

Nutritional value per serving: 70 Calories; 3.4g Fat; 5.1g Carbs; 2.4g Protein; 1.8g Sugars

Ingredients

- 1 cup chocolate chunks, sugar-free
- 3 tablespoons cocoa powder
- 3/4 cup buttermilk
- 1/2 cup milk
- 2 tablespoons whiskey
-

- 1/4 teaspoon grated nutmeg
- 1/8 teaspoon ground cloves
- 1/8 teaspoon cinnamon powder
- 1/2 teaspoon vanilla paste

Directions

1. Melt chocolate, along with cocoa and buttermilk in a microwave-safe bowl, on high for 70 seconds.
2. Stir in the other ingredients. Pour the mixture into silicone molds.

3. Refrigerate at least 1 hour 30 minutes. Bon appétit!

119. Vanilla Walnut Cheesecake

Preparation Time:1 hour

Servings:14

Nutritional value per serving: 393 Calories; 38g Fat; 4.1g Carbs; 9.8g Protein; 0.4g Sugars

Ingredients

- 8 ounces walnuts, chopped
- 8 packets stevia
- 1/4 teaspoon grated nutmeg
- A pinch of salt
- 1/2 cup butter, melted
- For the Filling:
- 22 ounces cream cheese, at room temperature
- 30 packets stevia
- 4 eggs
- 1 teaspoon vanilla essence
- 1 teaspoon pure almond extract
- 14 ounces sour cream

Directions

1. Combine all ingredients for the crust until well mixed; press the crust mixture into a springform pan. Set aside

2. Now, beat cream cheese on low speed until creamy and fluffy.

3. Add stevia and eggs, one at a time; mix on low speed. Add the remaining ingredients until well mixed.

4. Bake in the preheated oven at 300 degrees F for 55 minutes. Let it cool on a wire rack. Serve well chilled.

21-DAY MEAL PLAN

DAY	BREAKFAST	LUNCH	DINNER	DESSERT
1	Pizza Dip	Wrapped and Grilled Salmon with Saffron	Easy Pork Roast Casserole	Cheesy Coconut Cake
2	Mexican Breakfast	One Pan Chicken Mix	Chicken and Parsnips	Coconut Apple Cobbler
3	Feta Omelet	Lunch Caesar Salad	Pork and Bacon Baked Casserole	Easy Almond Fudge
4	Morning Pie	Sour and Spicy Spareribs	Meatloaf with Gruyere	Peanut Ice Cream
5	Sausage Patties	Lemon Salmon and Broccoli Casserole	Beef Stroganoff	Coconut Chia Pudding
6	Breakfast Mix	Broccoli Croquets	Pork with Button Mushrooms Casserole	Festive Cake with Cream Cheese Frosting
7	Sausage Quiche	Kaula" Pork with Cabbage	Simple "Grilled" Shrimp	Sinfully Delicious Whiskey Chocolate Bites
8	Eggplant Stew	Smoked Salmon Salad	Chinese Chicken Soup	Cheesy Coconut Cake
9	Chicken Omelet	Zucchini Wraps with the Cream Cheese	Wrapped and Grilled Salmon with Saffron	Summer Frappe Dessert
10	Kale Fritters	Chicken Salad	Braised Sour Pork Filet	heesecake Cupcakes with Vanilla

				Frosting
11	Italian Spaghetti Casserole	Baked Sea Bass with Fresh Herbs	Chicken and Leeks Mix	Vanilla Walnut Cheesecake
12	Cream Cheese Soufflé	Tender Pork Shoulder with Hot Peppers	Pork with Button Mushrooms Casserole	Lemon Lilliputian Fat Bombs
13	Morning Casserole	Herbed Shrimp with Cilantro	Parisian Schnitzel	Chilly Tuna Fat Balls
14	Breakfast Bread	Chicken and Leeks MixIFI	Parisian Schnitzel	Coconut Chia Pudding
15	Morning Pie	Apple Salad	Chicken and Mango Chutney	Coconut Apple Cobbler
16	Breakfast Mix	Indian Chicken Soup	Coconut Stew	Pork Rind Puppy Chow
17	Sausage Quiche	Bok Choy Salad	Braised Sour Pork Filet	Easy Rutabaga Fries
18	Cream Cheese Soufflé	Sour and Spicy Spareribs	Chicken and Leeks Mix	Dilled Chicken Wingettes with Goat Cheese Dip
19	Sausage Patties	Chicken and Parsnips	Sour and Spicy Spareribs	Cheese, Ham and Greek Yogurt
20	Pizza Dip	Halloumi Salad	Tender Pork Shoulder with Hot Peppers	Cocktail Salad on a Stick
21	Feta Omelet	Chicken and Parsnips	Simple "Grilled" Shrimp	Celery Root French Fries with Pine Nuts

TOP INTERMITTENT FASTING TIPS

Fasting proficiency only comes with experience. The more you actively use fasting for weight loss, the better you get at it. This is true both for how your body gets used to it and for how you get used to making the necessary choices. Even the smallest, most insignificant choice you make can have profound effects on the success of your fast. Fasting is a long experiment into trial and error. Thankfully, you don't have to repeat the same mistakes that others have done in the past. Below are some of the major tips you may need to use to enhance your intermittent fasting journey.

Taking Inventory of Your Medical and Eating Habits

Not everyone should be fasting, period. Some people want to shove fasting into their busy lives with no regards for how it will play out. People who are already used to eating clean, or clean enough will have the least amount of issues making the transition. However, for those who are pleasure eaters and regularly consume refined carbs and sugar, it can be a nightmare. Detoxifying from these types of diets will cause significant stress to the liver and will exacerbate the negative symptoms of the fast.

Talk with Your Doctor or Dietitian Before Making the Switch

There is no wrong way to do a fast, except if you do it without consulting a medical professional first. If you are already experiencing health issues, then it becomes doubly important. Choosing a more strenuous fasting routine necessitates that you undergo more medical supervision.

DON'T Assume That Fasting Will Fit into Your Lifestyle

Let's face it, skipping meals and drinking nothing but water all day is still uncharted waters for the majority of the population. It's weird, quirky and even controversial for many. Our lifestyles are defined by the combination of things we do and the people we interact with the most. Both of these things can and will get in the way of a poorly programmed fasting routine. Do you regularly eat out with our significant other or the people at work? Problem. Do you take your kids out for meals? Problem. Is your work schedule demanding and stress inducing? And if so are you a stress eater? Problem

Have a Serious Conversation with Yourself About the Changes Your Lifestyle Can Afford

The best way to confront rigid lifestyles is to single out the most pressing problem areas and see what you can do about it. Compromise is the key to success. Talk with those who you are closest with about your plans to lose weight. How can they support you on your journey? Sometimes, this will mean shopping and cooking for yourself and hiding the snacks. Your partner shouldn't feel obligated to follow your diet with you, but they should at least be supportive throughout.

Never Start a Fast Like It Was Just Another Thing You Do

It is a good thing to become comfortable with your fasting routines, but too much comfort is a bad thing. You start to get lazy and gradually start introducing changes that you were completely against in the beginning. This may mean allowing yourself to drink a diet soda on a Water Fast. Or it may mean ending your fasts a little earlier because "something came up."

Prepare Yourself Mentally, Take Note of Personal Boundaries, and Make Rituals

A fast should be a systemic habit that you do with the end goal always in mind. Fasting can be draining, and because of it, people get lazy and start to allow things. Mentally preparing yourself can be as easy as repeating the goals of the fast at every interval along the way. Before finishing your last meal, repeat for how long the fast will last and what you are allowed to eat. Do this upon waking up as well. To increase mental preparedness, create rituals to go with your fasts. Do you skip breakfast every fasting day? Maybe you read the daily newspaper on a park bench or give the bathroom a quick rub down instead. Rituals will help make the fast go by faster and form patterns in your mind.

Never Treat Your Fasting Routines Like a Competition Against Yourself

Having the resolve to push a fast through completion is necessary for success, but it can work against you. There are times when weight loss becomes such an integral part of our being that we convince ourselves that we must do all in our power to attain our goals. Unfortunately, fasting doesn't work that way. Fasting is a numbers game. Even if you miss one or two fasts here and there but keep doing it regularly, results will always be in your favor

Listen to Your Body and Throw in the Towel When Necessary

Ultimately, it is your body that decides whether you should go through with a fast or not. Listen to your body carefully. Understand what the symptoms are for low-blood sugar episodes. There is no rush to the finish line, only being in harmony with your mind and body.

CONCLUSION

Thanks for downloading this book. It's my firm belief that it has provided you with all the answers to your questions.

Intermittent fasting is more of a lifestyle than it is a diet. It is an ancient rejoinder to our modern, highly saturated lives that gravitate towards the excess. Fasting is simple, easy, and effective. You don't have to be a spiritual ascetic to enjoy the pleasures of fasting, either. It is both a way to challenge yourself and to cleanse your body from the toxic food that you eat.

Your fitness journey doesn't have to end at simple weight loss. Losing weight is one thing—looking and feeling good is another. The next logical step after reaching your weight loss goals is to gain lean mass in a healthy fashion. Intermittent fasting will help you keep the fat down. Meanwhile, strength training exercises will pack on the muscle. A higher percentage of lean mass means that you will fit into clothes better and that your self-confidence will soar.

45297962R00075